THE AMERICAN DIETETIC ASSOCIATION

W9-ARI-347

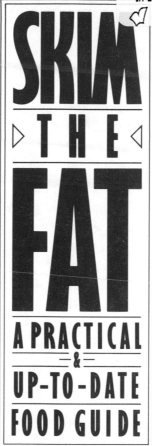

SKIM ▷THE◁ FAT

A PRACTICAL
—&—
UP-TO-DATE
FOOD GUIDE

The American Dietetic Association is the largest group of food and nutrition professionals in the world. As the advocate of the profession, the ADA serves the public by promoting optimal nutrition, health, and well-being.

For expert answers to your nutrition questions, call the ADA/National Center for Nutrition and Dietetics Hot Line at (800) 366-1655, and speak directly with a registered dietitian (RD), listen to recorded messages, or obtain a referral to an RD in your area.

JOHN WILEY & SONS, INC.

New York • Chichester • Weinheim • Brisbane • Singapore • Toronto

The information contained in this book is not intended to serve as a replacement for
professional medical advice. Any use of the information in this book is at the reader's
discretion. The author and the publisher specifically disclaim any and all liability arising
directly or indirectly from the use or application of any information contained in this
book. A health care professional should be consulted regarding your specific situation.

ISBN 0-471-34703-5

Printed in the United States of America

10   9   8   7   6   5   4   3   2

Contents

Skim the Fat

* Some of the recipes in this section are from *The Healthy Weigh: A Practical Food Guide*, published by The American Dietetic Association, 1991. Other recipes were created by The American Dietetic Association for the April 1995 issue of *Ladies Home Journal*.

Introduction

Skim the Fat
A Practical Food Guide

The fact that Americans eat too much fat, particularly saturated fat, is not news. A number of reports on diet and health clearly indicate that fat makes up close to 40 percent of the total calories in many people's diets. The trouble with this high-fat eating style is that it can set the stage for health problems.

Studies show that a diet too high in fat may increase the risk for many lifestyle-related illnesses, including heart disease, stroke, high blood pressure, obesity, and certain types of cancer.

Although dozens of books offer suggestions on how to lower the fat, most people find themselves bogged down in a sea of confusing fat terms. Which fat is "good"? Which fat is "bad"? How much fat is too much?

Skim the Fat: A Practical Food Guide helps to clear up these issues with a short, to-the-point approach to dealing with fat. Along with explanations about why fat is a necessary nutrient come specific guidelines about how much and what type of fat to eat.

The main focus of this book is practicality. Brief charts, tables, and text offer quick, usable bits of information about the fat content of foods. Low-fat recipes are also included to help you put fat knowledge into practice.

Skim the Fat

Chapter 1

Figuring Out Fats

Why bother to figure out fats? Well, for starters, because we know the following:

▲ Excess fat intake can raise cholesterol levels and increase the risk of heart disease and stroke.

▲ Excess fat intake may increase the risk for some types of cancer, particularly of the colon, prostate, or breast.

▲ Excess fat, especially saturated fat, has been linked with high blood pressure, regardless of a person's body weight.

▲ Excess fat may increase the risk for diabetes.

▲ Excess fat is likely to make people fat because each gram of fat has nine calories, compared with four calories for each gram of carbohydrate or protein.

Nonetheless, fat is a nutrient, and your body does need some fat to maintain your good health and nutrition. Which raises another question: What exactly are we talking about when we use the word nutrition?

Nutrition is the science or study of the proper balance of food to promote good health. The fundamental activities of the human body, such as the intake of food, digestion, release of energy, elimination of wastes, and the use of nutrients essential for maintenance, growth, and reproduction are all part of the study of nutrition.

The foods you eat must contain, in adequate amounts, about 45 to 50 highly important substances essential to sustain life. These are in addition to water and oxygen. These substances are known as nutrients.

Nutrients

The essential nutrients are proteins, carbohydrate, fats, vitamins, and minerals.

The human body also needs dietary fiber, which aids in the efficient elimination of waste products from the body.

The basic nutrients—protein, carbohydrate, and fat, plus the vitamins and minerals—and fiber should all be available to us through the food we eat. If we are obtaining all that we need by eating the appropriate variety of foods, we should not need to take any additional nutritional supplements.

But just how do we make sure we get all that we need from the foods we eat? And, since fat is one of the big three on that nutrient list, just how much fat do we actually need?

The Facts About Fat

Fat helps maintain healthy skin and hair; it transports fat-soluble vitamins through the blood, and it regulates cholesterol levels. It also stores the body's excess calories.

All fats have the same number of calories per gram, but the fats themselves are not all the same.

If you want to follow a heart-healthy diet, for example, you'll want to cut back on the amount of highly *saturated* fats you consume. These are most abundant in foods like lard, butter, fat in meats, coconut oil, palm kernel oil, fat in cheese, and solid shortenings. On the other hand, diets containing *monounsaturated fats*— like olive, canola, and peanut oils—seem to promote heart health.

Fat has traditionally been seen as the "bad guy." This is understandable since it has been linked to obesity, heart disease, and cancer. But some fat is necessary for good health. It is the amount and the type of fat we eat that gets us into trouble. And that is essentially what this book is about.

Fat, as we said, is a nutrient. And like any other nutrient it performs vital functions in the body.

▲ Fat is a building block for some chemicals that help the body work.

▲ Fat also cushions and protects vital organs.

▲ Fat acts as a storage facility for fat-soluble vitamins.

Despite these critical functions, the body doesn't need large quantities of fat. And that's part of the problem.

Fats provide nine calories of energy per gram, more than twice the energy in carbohydrates or proteins. It's easy to see how people can gain weight by eating too many high-fat foods.

Excess fat calories are stored as body fat. But the fact that too much fat can cause obesity is only part of the story. Too much of the wrong kind of fat can create other health problems.

Kinds of Fat

There are three major types of fat in foods:

▲ saturated

▲ monounsaturated

▲ polyunsaturated

It's not necessary to learn chemistry to understand these dietary fats. All you need to remember is that some saturated fats—concentrated in animal foods like meats, whole milk, and butter—raise blood cholesterol levels. Polyunsaturated vegetable fats, like corn oil and safflower oil, and monounsaturated fats, like olive oil, do just the opposite. That sounds like a simple enough concept. But to understand the idea better, it helps to become familiar with some of the terms related to fats, such as saturated and unsaturated fat, cholesterol, and trans fatty acids, which can sometimes be very confusing.

What's So Important About Saturated Fat?

Saturated fat is an abbreviation of the term *saturated fatty acids*. Although all foods contain a mixture of saturated and unsaturated fatty acids, higher concentrations of one type of fat are more likely to be found.

Animal foods like meats, whole milk, cream, and cheese are high in saturated fat. Olive oil and fish contain higher levels of unsaturated fats.

Small amounts of saturated fat in the diet are not harmful. (The Dietary Guidelines for Americans recommend limiting saturated fat to less than 10 percent of total calories, or one third of the total fat intake.) But eating too much saturated fat can raise blood cholesterol levels.

Most saturated fats tend to be solid at room temperature. Manufacturers may process liquid vegetable oils into hydrogenated oils or solid shortenings to improve baking qualities and extend shelf life. The end product is not only more saturated but also more solid than the original oil.

Prime Sources of Saturated Fat

Butter

Cheese

Whole milk

Cream

Meat

Poultry

Chocolate

Coconut

Coconut oil

Palm oil

Palm kernel oil

Lard

Other solid shortenings

What's So Important About Unsaturated Fat?

Unsaturated fats fall into two categories: *monounsaturated* and *polyunsaturated*. Again, the terms refer to monounsaturated fatty acids and polyunsaturated fatty acids.

> Taking the skin off chicken, draining the fat from cooked hamburger, and using skim milk are all ways to cut back on the amount of saturated fat you eat.

Monounsaturated fats are found in peanuts, olives, olive oil, and canola oil. Reports from Mediterranean countries like Greece and Italy, where the incidence of certain kinds of disease is rare, suggest that a diet rich in monounsaturated fats may help lessen the risk for heart disease.

Polyunsaturated fats, which are found commonly in many vegetable foods, also appear to be healthful for the heart.

Studies show that when these fats replace saturated fats, they are capable of lowering the level of cholesterol in the blood. Vegetable oils like corn oil, safflower oil, and soybean oil are examples of polyunsaturated fats.

Cholesterol

Animal products are the source of all dietary cholesterol. Eating less fat from animal sources will help lower cholesterol as well as total fat and saturated fat in your diet.

Keep in mind, however, that all goals for fats apply to the diet over several days, not a single meal or food. Some foods that contain fat, saturated fat, and cholesterol, such as meats, milk, cheese, and eggs, also

Prime Sources of Monounsaturated Fat

Olives

Olive oil

Peanuts

Peanut oil

Avocados

Canola oil

Cashews

Prime Sources of Polyunsaturated Fat

Corn oil

Cottonseed oil

Sunflower oil

Safflower oil

Soybean oil

Soft margarine

Fish

contain high-quality protein and are our best sources for certain vitamins and minerals. Low-fat choices of these foods are lean meat and low-fat milk and cheeses.

What About Fish Oils?

Omega-3 fatty acids are polyunsaturated fatty acids and are components of the oil found in fish. Some studies show that eating fish with omega-3 fatty acids several times a week lowers blood cholesterol and triglyceride (another fat) levels in the bloodstream.

Good sources of omega-3 fatty acids include cold-water marine fish such as salmon, tuna, haddock, mackerel, sea trout, and herring. Other fish contain omega-3 fatty acids in much lesser amounts. Fish oil supplements are not recommended for a variety of reasons. All the nutrients, vitamins, and minerals are much more efficiently absorbed when they are derived from food sources.

Fitting Fats and Oils Into Your Diet

To make vegetable oils more versatile, they are often hardened by a process called hydrogenation. During the hydrogenation process, some of the fats are changed to become trans fatty acids. Trans fatty acids also occur naturally in beef, pork, lamb, butter, and milk. There is little scientific evidence to suggest that current consumption levels of trans fatty acids need to be changed.

Health professionals agree, however, that reducing total fat and saturated fat intake are the most important dietary changes you can make to promote better health. Whether you are trying to find a healthy weight, lower cholesterol levels, or just eat a healthful diet, focus on reducing total fat.

MYTHS & MISCONCEPTIONS

ABOUT FAT AND CHOLESTEROL

Myth

Eliminate red meats
if a healthy heart
is your goal.

Fact: Plenty of lean cuts of beef and pork are low in fat. Furthermore, red meat is an excellent source of both iron and zinc.

Action: Choose "select" grades of beef instead of fattier "prime" or "choice" cuts. Opt for moderate portions of the leanest cuts: eye of round, top round, tenderloin. Use lean cooking methods such as broiling, baking, and roasting.

Myth

Margarine has fewer
calories than butter.

Fact: Both fats have the same number of calories. The advantage of margarine is that it has less saturated fat than butter and no cholesterol. Butter-margarine blends fall somewhere in between.

Action: Choose margarine as an everyday fat; tub margarine is less saturated than stick.

Myth

It makes little difference
which low-fat milk
you drink.

Fact: Skim milk is much lower in fat than 1%, 2%, or whole milk. One 8-ounce glass of skim milk has less than 1 gram of fat; 1% milk carries 2.4 grams, and 2% contains 4.7 grams.

Action: Gradually wean yourself away from 2% milk, if you can, by mixing it with 1%; use skim milk in cooking.

Myth

There are good fats and bad fats, and the bad fats are best avoided.

Fact: The story is not so simple. Most foods contain a mixture of saturated, polyunsaturated, and monounsaturated fats. The idea is to strike a balance among all three types. Saturated fats, since they raise blood cholesterol levels, should account for no more than one third of the fat total.

Action: Focus efforts on cutting back on total fat. Allow for some saturated fats, but choose more often from the list of polyunsaturated and monounsaturated fats.

Chapter 2

How Much Fat Can I Eat?

It's a legitimate question. We do need some fat, but just exactly how much?

Some years back, the U.S. government recommended that Americans aim for 30 percent or less of daily calories from fat. The average intake at that time was about 40 percent.

That means if you consume 1800 calories in a day—the amount recommended for an active woman who weighs 130 pounds—540 calories, or 30 percent, can come from fat. That's the equivalent of 14 teaspoons of fat, or 60 grams per day. Stated in teaspoons, it seems like a lot, but because so much of the fat we eat is "hidden" in foods, the grams add up quickly.

For years, researchers have been producing graphs showing high rates of cancer and heart disease in countries consuming large amounts of high-fat foods. Once Japanese people started eating more western-style foods, they started showing an increase in the incidence of these diseases, too.

Today, health experts agree that less than 30 percent of your total daily calories should come from fat, with the right balance probably being a one-third, one-third, one-third split among saturated, monounsaturated, and polyunsaturated fats. Keep in mind that it's not necessary to track how many grams of each type of fat you eat each day. Instead, by learning a few basic facts about the sources of each type of fat, you can learn to average.

If you choose fat from a variety of food sources, you will be able to keep a good balance. Your first strategy, however, is to cut back on total fat.

Figuring Out What Your Body Needs

Height and weight charts tell us something about how much we may want to weigh at a given height. The following chart adjusts the weight goals by age. The higher weights in the ranges generally apply to men who tend to have more muscle than bone; the lower weights apply to women.

Suggested Weights* (in Pounds) for Adults		
Height	Ages 19 to 34 years	Ages 35 and older
5'0"	97-128	108-138
5'1"	101-132	111-143
5'2"	104-137	115-148
5'3"	107-141	119-152
5'4"	111-146	122-157
5'5"	114-150	126-162
5'6"	118-155	130-167
5'7"	121-160	134-172
5'8"	125-164	138-178
5'9"	129-169	142-183
5'10"	132-174	146-188
5'11"	136-179	151-194
6'0"	140-184	155-199
6'1"	144-189	159-205
6'2"	148-195	164-210
6'3"	152-200	168-216
6'4"	156-205	173-222
6'5"	160-211	177-228
6'6"	164-216	182-234

*Weight without shoes and clothing.

Source: Derived from National Research Council, 1989.

Calculating Your Calories

In addition to weight, daily activity levels need to be considered in determining daily calorie needs.

The following formula helps to determine the number of daily calories it takes to maintain your current weight. The formula gives you a "ballpark" figure and will vary from person to person, depending on levels of activity, the amount of muscle versus fat in the body, and age.

Multiply your current weight in pounds   (_____)

     by 10 if you are inactive
     by 12 if you are moderately active
     by 15 if you are extremely active

This number equals the calories needed for the day to maintain your current weight.   (_____)

Now, let's try the formula again using your desired weight from the chart on page 10.

Multiply your desired weight in pounds   (_____)

     by 10 if you are inactive
     by 12 if you are moderately active
     by 15 if you are extremely active

This equals the number of calories you need each day to maintain your desired weight.   (_____)

If you want to reach your desired weight on the chart, strive to eat the number of calories allowed for that weight. This formula, even though simple, takes into account weight, activity levels, and the required energy to sustain them.

A Thirty-Percent Solution

When health experts first suggested that 30 percent or less of a person's total calories should come from fat, the recommendation seemed pretty straight forward. The problem, however, is that many people assume that the 30 percent rule applies to every single food they eat. In truth, the 30 percent number is meant to be a daily average.

Say you eat a food that contains 50 percent of its 100 calories from fat—a homemade chocolate chip cookie, for example. To offset that higher fat level, you could choose to eat more fruits, vegetables, or other low-fat foods at other times that day.

Health experts stress the importance of being flexible with high- and low-fat food choices. There is no reason for people to deny themselves foods they enjoy. A few potato chips, an occasional slice of cheesecake, or a pastrami sandwich won't destroy an otherwise low-fat diet. But, work for balance. If you have high-fat foods, find the low-fat foods that will compensate and help you keep within the 30 percent guideline.

Fat Balancing

Another way to look at the advice to eat 30 percent or less of calories from fat is to convert that percentage into total grams of fat per day, based on how many calories you eat. It's just another way of coming up with a healthy fat balance.

Scientists from the United States Department of Agriculture (USDA) estimate that 1600 calories per day is an adequate level for many sedentary women and older adults.

Most children, teenage girls, and active women probably need about 2200 calories per day to fuel body activities. Teenage boys and many active men can require as much as 2800 calories or more per day.

The chart that follows uses some typical calorie levels and converts the recommendation for 30 percent fat into grams of fat.

Now that most foods in supermarkets are nutritionally labeled, it is much easier to keep track of fat grams in many of the foods you eat.

Keep in mind that it's not necessary to count out the grams of fat you eat each day. But this method of fat balancing provides a starting point for helping you assess current fat intake. Then every once in a while, you can check up on yourself to make sure your diet stays low in fat.

If you eat . . .	allow yourself up to . . .
1200 calories	40 grams of fat per day
1500 calories	50 grams of fat per day
1800 calories	60 grams of fat per day
2100 calories	70 grams of fat per day
2400 calories	80 grams of fat per day
2600 calories	87 grams of fat per day
2800 calories	93 grams of fat per day

Where Does Cholesterol Fit Into This Fat Picture?

Cholesterol is not a fat, but a waxy, fat-like substance. Cholesterol is found only in foods of animal origin. Meat, poultry, fish, milk, cheese, egg yolks, and organ meats are all food sources of cholesterol. No plant foods contain cholesterol.

Studies show that eating cholesterol-rich foods can raise the blood cholesterol level in some people, increasing their risk for heart disease. However, cholesterol-rich foods don't have as strong an impact on blood cholesterol levels as saturated fat. Still, the American Heart Association advises Americans to limit cholesterol in the diet to no more than 300 milligrams per day.

One egg yolk contains 213 milligrams of cholesterol, or two-thirds of the daily limit. For this reason, experts recommend setting a limit of three or four egg yolks per week. Organ meats, such as liver, are also high in cholesterol. The chart on page 33 contains more information about the cholesterol content of various foods.

If this all sounds very complicated, just remember that a diet low in total fat and saturated fat is also likely to fall within the recommended range for cholesterol.

What's Your Fat IQ ?

Advice to eat lean meats, whole grains, and vegetables isn't much help when real-life situations call for choices that don't fit into those categories. What snack do you munch on at coffee break? What type of pie will do the least fat damage? Here are a few fat puzzlers that confront most of us at one time or another.

See if you can select the lowest-fat item from each of these groups.

1. Breakfast out: French toast, waffles, or pancakes?
2. Burrito topper: guacamole, salsa, or sour cream?
3. Sandwich filler: tuna salad, roast beef, or ham and cheese?
4. Italian main course: eggplant parmigiana, spaghetti with marinara sauce, or lasagna?
5. Frozen treat: fruit bar, fudge ice milk bar, or frozen yogurtt bar?
6. Morning bread: glazed doughnut, bagel, or croissant?
7. Breakfast meat: bacon, Canadian bacon, or turkey sausage?
8. Afternoon work break: microwave popcorn, pretzels, or potato chips?
9. Pie plate: lemon chiffon, apple, pumpkin, or pecan?

Turn the page for the answers!

Answers

1. Pick the pancake. Two 4-inch rounds typically carry only 2 to 3 grams of fat. One slice of French toast has 6 to 7 grams of fat, and a large homemade waffle carries about 8 to 13 grams. (Toaster waffles weigh in with 2 to 5 grams each.)

2. Stick with salsa. Chopped tomatoes, vegetables, and salsa spices are virtually fat free. Guacamole, made from avocado, is high in fat. (One avocado carries 30 grams of fat.) Two tablespoons of sour cream have 5 grams of fat.

3. Can you believe it, the roast beef wins on total fat content with just 10 to 13 grams of fat, although it does carry more saturated fat than tuna. But the tuna salad has almost twice the total fat (from mayonnaise) in just a 1/2 cup serving. Ham and cheese fits somewhere in the middle. (Note: These numbers are for modest-size sandwiches; deli sandwiches piled high with meat and cheese are a different story.)

4. Any kind of plain pasta with marinara (red) sauce is a good choice. Both the parmigiana (lots of cheese, fried eggplant) and lasagna (usually three types of cheese and plenty of meat) can carry 20 or more grams of fat per serving. Ditto for spaghetti with meatballs.

5. Believe it or not, these treats are all lean. Frozen fruit bars, except for the coconut variety, contain no fat. Fudge ice milk bars weigh in with just 2 grams; yogurt bars typically carry 2 to 4 grams.

6. Reach for the plain bagel. A bagel sports a mere 2 grams of fat. Even if you add a teaspoon of margarine (4 grams of fat), it still amounts to far less than the 11 grams of fat in a yeast doughnut or croissant. Spread the bagel with fruit jam (no fat) for an even lower fat total.

7. Canadian bacon wins by a long shot. One slice contains less than 2 grams of fat. A similar size portion of bacon (3 crisp slices) has nearly 10 grams. One link of turkey sausage falls in between at 5 grams of fat.

8. Munch on the pretzels. They have only a trace of fat and no cholesterol. More than half of the calories of both potato chips and microwave popcorn come from pure fat. However, some of the "light" microwave popcorns contain as little as 1 gram of fat, instead of the 5 to 12 grams per 3-cup portion of the regular versions.

9. The lemon chiffon (10 grams of fat), apple (12 grams of fat), and pumpkin (13 grams of fat) are much better than the pecan (24 grams of fat). Because of the nuts, the pecan pie has more than twice the fat of the lemon chiffon.

Skim the Fat

Chapter 3

What You Need to Know About Fat and Heart Disease

Heart disease is the nation's number one killer, and even as researchers continue to look for ways to prevent the devastating toll this illness takes on Americans, there's little doubt that a diet high in fat helps set the stage for heart disease.

But diet is only one factor that can influence your risk for heart disease.

Other major risk factors include:

▲ cigarette smoking

▲ high blood pressure

▲ high blood cholesterol

▲ family history of coronary heart disease

▲ being male

▲ diabetes

▲ sedentary lifestyle

▲ obesity

Special Concerns

Each of these risk factors alone can increase the chances that you will get heart disease. In other words, a high blood cholesterol level can increase heart disease risk all by itself. But you should know that when high blood cholesterol is combined with another risk factor (say high blood pressure or cigarette smoking), risk for heart disease escalates dramatically.

For example, if your cholesterol level is more than 240 milligrams per deciliter (mg./dL.) and you also have high blood pressure, your risk for heart disease can be six times greater than if you had neither of these risk factors.

Diet and Heart Disease

The high-fat American diet is a major culprit in heart disease, no question. Eating cholesterol-rich foods increases blood cholesterol levels. Eating large amounts of saturated fats, the kind found in meat and whole-fat dairy products, promotes the production of cholesterol in the body. Those are the facts.

The antidote? Eat a low-fat, high-fiber diet of fruits, vegetables, and whole grains, with omega-3 fatty acids from fish like mackerel, salmon, and fresh tuna. In addition, fill up on foods like broccoli, carrots, and citrus fruits, all of which add their own special protection as antioxidants.

Besides diet, you can reduce your risks by stopping smoking, reading the next chapter on how to control blood cholesterol levels, increasing the amount of physical activity in your life, and losing weight if you need to.

These principles apply whether you are a man, a woman, or a child. Indeed, experts want Americans to realize that no one is immune to heart disease. In fact, researchers now single out various age and population groups with specific messages about their heart disease risk.

For Women Only

While it's true that genetics give women a slight edge when it comes to heart disease risk, that edge all but disappears after menopause. So why not wait until then to be concerned?

Experts say that lifestyle factors—smoking, obesity, inactivity— can still take a toll on women in early years. A woman who smokes will damage her heart despite the fact that other protective factors are at work. If she quits smoking, her risk for heart disease drops by about 50 percent. The health message for women: Don't be complacent about heart disease. It can happen to anyone.

Childhood Concerns

For a number of years the subject of children and cholesterol was fraught with controversy. Then the National Cholesterol Education Program (NCEP) issued cholesterol guidelines for children.

Basically, the diet advice is the same as for adults. However, parents should not start moderating their children's fat intake until after age two. Before that time, fat and cholesterol are crucial for healthy cell and brain development.

What about cholesterol testing? The NCEP committee says testing in children is unwarranted unless the family has a history of heart disease.

Because diet and exercise patterns are established in youth, it is particularly important for parents to move their children away from a high-fat diet and a sedentary lifestyle toward a lower fat diet and an active life.

Infants and toddlers less than two years old, as stated earlier, need a diet high in cholesterol and fat. About half the calories in mother's milk come from fat, and saturated fatty acids make up almost half of those calories.

Cow's milk and infant formula are also high in fat, but they contain a different mix of fatty acids than mother's milk. Cow's milk, for example, has more saturated fatty acids, less monounsaturated fatty acids, and much less polyunsaturated fatty acids. In contrast, infant formulas are higher in polyunsaturated fatty acids but contain virtually no cholesterol.

Infants respond to high-fat, high-cholesterol milk in the same way that adults would. Their serum cholesterol levels are raised. But most health experts believe this should be no cause for concern. Children are breastfed or take formula for only a short period of time, so the high cholesterol level probably has no lasting effects. Perhaps even more important, however, breast milk, in particular, meets other nutritional needs of infants. Thus, parents should not try to reduce the amount of fat their infants and toddlers consume.

But that is not the case with children once they start eating the same foods as adults. The consequences of having high serum cholesterol as a child are not yet clear, but two pieces of evidence suggest that the outcome may not be good.

▲ Children with high cholesterol levels tend to become teenagers and young adults with high cholesterol.

▲ In addition, doctors have found that significant numbers of young adults already have detectable atherosclerosis, the condition that results from cholesterol deposits on artery walls.

Therefore it seems that children older than two years have as much to gain from reducing their fat intake as do adults.

Some people have questioned the safety of tampering with our children's diets. After all, our children are far healthier today than they were at the beginning of this century, thanks in part to improved nutrition. But many studies show that a moderate-fat diet is safe for children. These studies show, too, that there is no need for healthy people over the age of two to get more than 30 percent of their calories from fat.

Cholesterol After Age 65

What can you do about preventing heart disease in your senior years? Isn't it a little too late to start making changes in diet and lifestyle?

Definitely not. Data from the Honolulu heart study—a large medical investigation of nearly 1500 men over the age of 65—show that high blood cholesterol levels are linked with higher heart disease risk. In other words, high blood cholesterol levels are just as risky at 65 as at 25.

Having a heart attack or stroke in later years can cause disability and diminish quality of life. That is why it pays to keep tabs on cholesterol and health no matter what your age.

High Blood Pressure

High blood pressure is also on the list of variables that influence your risk for heart disease. Blood pressure measures the force exerted by blood against the arterial wall.

The top number measures the systolic pressure, which is generated when the heart contracts and pushes blood into the arteries. The bottom number measures the diastolic pressure, or the pressure of the arteries when the heart muscle relaxes between beats.

Normal blood pressure is 120/80. Pressures over that number are considered borderline high. One in six American adults has high blood pressure—that is, a systolic pressure over 140 and a diastolic pressure over 90. Even a slightly elevated blood pressure can increase the risk of having a heart attack or stroke and should not be ignored.

Being overweight increases the odds that you will develop high blood pressure. Therefore, maintaining a healthful weight is essential. Food can also play a role in helping to keep your blood pressure within normal limits.

Omega-3 fatty acids, for example, which are found in salmon, fresh albacore tuna, and sardines, lower the levels of thromboxane, a substance that is produced by the body and causes blood vessels to constrict. Elevated thromboxane levels are linked to high blood pressure.

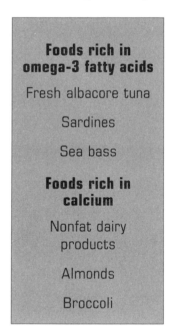

Foods rich in omega-3 fatty acids

Fresh albacore tuna

Sardines

Sea bass

Foods rich in calcium

Nonfat dairy products

Almonds

Broccoli

A study from the Harvard School of Public Health showed that people who ate a diet high in fruit fiber had lower systolic blood pressures than people who did not. Other forms of fiber were not found to be significant.

Additionally, the study showed that higher levels of magnesium intake were associated with lower levels of blood pressure. Magnesium is also found in fruits and vegetables.

Other foods have been found to lower blood pressure as well, including garlic and cruciferous vegetables like broccoli and cabbage, and citrus fruits. The Framingham Children's Study (Framingham, Massachusetts) found that children who ate the most calcium-rich foods had the lowest systolic pressures.

Sodium chloride, or table salt, can raise blood pressure in salt-sensitive people.

Diabetes

Diabetes is also on the list of risk factors for heart disease. In fact, diabetes mellitus is an umbrella term used to describe several different but related metabolic disorders that afflict up to 14 million Americans.

These diabetes-related disorders are the seventh leading cause of death in the United States. Women are nearly twice as likely to develop diabetes as men. If untreated, diabetes can lead to serious complications including heart attack, stroke, kidney disease, and blindness.

In general, diabetic disorders are characterized by hyperglycemia or high concentrations of glucose in the blood. The abnormally high glucose concentrations may be caused by an inadequate amount of insulin (the hormone that gets blood glucose into body cells where it fuels many important body functions) or by the body's inability to respond properly to the insulin it produces, which is known as insulin resistance.

Type I or insulin-dependent diabetes (formerly called juvenile diabetes) is caused by the inability of the pancreas to produce any insulin at all. Type I diabetes usually strikes suddenly and dramatically before age 40. People with this form of diabetes must take insulin to maintain normal blood glucose levels.

Type II diabetes, also known as adult, non-insulin dependent, or late-onset diabetes, accounts for 90 percent of all cases of diabetes and occurs during or after middle age. Very often, there are no symptoms; typically a physician first detects the problem when a patient displays an elevated fasting blood glucose level after a routine physical.

There appears to be a genetic tendency to develop diabetes, although obesity is a major risk factor. In fact, between 80 and 90 percent of people with Type II diabetes are overweight.

Managing diabetes through proper meal planning can reduce your risk of complications such as heart disease, stroke, kidney disease or blindness. Such a plan should be designed especially for the person with diabetes by a registered dietitian. (See page 41 for more information about diabetes and diet.)

Obesity

Obesity is the last factor on the heart-disease-risk list. For more than 50 years, life insurance companies have pointed out that greatly increased body weight is associated with an above-average death rate.

In the course of investigating why this is so, researchers have developed a number of ways of judging whether people weigh more than they should for optimal health. The two most important factors associated with the risk of developing several chronic diseases are (1) total body fat, most often estimated by the ratio of body weight to height, and (2) distribution of that fat, on the stomach or on the hips and legs.

Where your body stores fat is the other clue to what makes a "healthy" weight. Excess body fat that settles around the middle, giving you a shape somewhat like an apple, puts you at higher risk for heart disease, high blood pressure, stroke, and diabetes. Excess weight that lodges below the waist, creating a pear-shaped body, does not appear to be as risky.

If the mirror doesn't tell you whether you are an apple or pear, use the following formula to determine your waist-to-hip ratio.

1. Stand relaxed, and measure your waist at its smallest point. Don't pull in your stomach.
2. Then measure your hips at the largest part of your buttocks.
3. Divide the waist measurement by the hip measurement. If the number is nearly 1.0, consider yourself an apple, and do something about losing those extra pounds.

Chapter 4

What Is a Healthy Blood Cholesterol Level?

Cholesterol, itself, is not bad. Actually, it is essential to life because it forms protective sheaths around nerves, helps make hormones and vitamin D, and combines with the bile acids that aid in the digestion of fat. We all need the right amount of cholesterol to maintain good health. However, too much cholesterol encourages the development of heart and blood vessel disease.

Cholesterol has been widely researched to determine what constitutes healthy or unhealthy levels because of its role in heart disease in humans. The logical next question is: How can we reduce cholesterol in our diets?

Cholesterol in Human Metabolism

Cholesterol is obtained by our bodies in two ways: from the liver, which manufactures it, and from the food we eat. The liver synthesizes enough cholesterol for all our body's needs—about 75 percent of the cholesterol in the average person's body (any we get from our food is actually extra). Our bodies can dispose of some extra cholesterol, but not all.

Cholesterol circulates through the bloodstream. It is a sterol, meaning it is not soluble in water, so the body combines it and other fats with protein to form complexes known as lipoproteins, which can be carried in the bloodstream.

There are two lipoproteins important to our discussion: high-density lipoproteins (HDL or the "healthy" lipoproteins) and low-density lipoproteins (LDL or the less desirable lipoproteins).

The high-density lipoproteins are often called "good cholesterol," because they carry cholesterol away from the body tissues and return it to the liver for recycling. The function of the low-density lipoproteins is to carry cholesterol to the cells where it can be deposited.

If the LDLs transport more cholesterol than the cells can use, the excess collects in the arteries. The LDL cholesterol then forms plaque, which builds up and produces the condition known as atherosclerosis. It is this buildup of plaque that is a precursor to heart attacks and strokes. For more information about atherosclerosis, see page 43.

The NCEP recommends that Americans keep their blood cholesterol levels below 200 mg./dL. Numbers lower than 200 equate with less risk for heart disease.

If a person's intake of dietary fat is high, many experts consider that levels of serum cholesterol will also increase, causing greater risk of heart disease and especially atherosclerosis. Studies have shown that high levels of HDL cholesterol reduce the risk of atherosclerosis, but high levels of other lipoproteins, particularly LDL, dramatically increase the risk.

There are some people whose bodies actually produce excessive amounts of cholesterol. These people, in particular, need to limit the amount of cholesterol and saturated fat they get from food. While various drugs can help lower cholesterol levels for persons with very high levels, experts still recommend that adults try to limit their cholesterol and saturated fat intake to reduce their overall risk of coronary disease.

How do you determine cholesterol level? Blood tests, preferably done in a hospital or medical clinic, are the most reliable measures of blood cholesterol levels. Mass screening (finger stick) cholesterol tests, such as those done at shopping malls, are not always accurate.

If a blood test shows that your cholesterol level is less than 200, you will not need testing for another five years. If a blood test shows that your cholesterol level is above 200, the doctor may order a lipid profile. These tests provide more specific information about the type of cholesterol in your blood.

Examining the Test Results

If you or a family member have a blood test to check total cholesterol levels, the figures below show you what number doctors and registered dietitians think is desirable. Look at the second set of figures if you have a lipoprotein analysis. Doctors will be concentrating not just on total blood cholesterol level, but also on the level of LDL cholesterol in the blood. Keep in mind that desirable levels in children are very different from those for adults.

Some Quick Facts about Cholesterol

▲ Levels of 140 to 180 are associated with the lowest rates of coronary heart disease.

▲ Levels of 180 to 200 are associated with substantially lower heart disease incidence and favorable overall health status.

▲ At 250 mg., the risk doubles over the risk at 200 mg.

▲ At 300 mg., the risk is four times higher than at 200 mg.

Diet is one of the first lines of defense against a high blood cholesterol level. Although the body produces its own supply of cholesterol, certain foods can contribute to the total. To better understand how food affects blood cholesterol, we need to understand the difference between blood cholesterol and dietary cholesterol.

Cholesterol Levels and Heart Disease Risk

Adults		Children*
Less than 200	Acceptable	Less than 170
200-239	Borderline-high	170-199
240 and above	High	200 & above

LDL Cholesterol Levels and Heart Disease Risk

Adults		Children*
Less than 130	Acceptable	Less than 110
130-159	Borderline-high	110-129
160 and above	High	130 & above

*Older than 2 years

(Data from "Reducing cholesterol in children and adolescents: a new report." National Heart, Lung, and Blood Institute Infomemo. July 1991. National Heart, Lung, and Blood Institute. Facts About Blood Cholesterol. Bethesda, Md: US Department of Health and Human Services, Public Health Service, National Institutes of Health, 1987.)

Dietary cholesterol is the cholesterol found in foods of animal origin, particularly egg yolks and organ meats. This cholesterol may influence your blood cholesterol level. But saturated fats, like those found in fatty meats, whole milk, and butter, raise the level of cholesterol in the blood even more.

Blood or serum cholesterol is the cholesterol that circulates in your blood. Your blood cholesterol levels reflect the cholesterol manufactured by your liver as well as the cholesterol coming from your diet.

What Is a Healthy Blood Cholesterol Level?

Because higher blood cholesterol levels are associated with a greater risk of heart disease, moderate consumption of dietary fat—especially saturated fat—and cholesterol could be beneficial to you and your heart. Obeying the general guidelines about fat in the pages that follow may help you ward off heart disease.

Because higher levels of HDLs, the "healthy" lipoproteins, may promote healthier arteries, the higher your HDLs, the lower your risk for developing heart disease. Recent studies suggest that HDL cholesterol even has the ability to remove plaque previously deposited on artery walls, thereby reversing atherosclerosis.

Here are some tips for how to raise your HDL levels:

▲ Limit your consumption of foods that are high in saturated fat and cholesterol.

▲ Engage in regular aerobic exercise.

▲ Stop smoking.

▲ Eat more fish (at least two or three times a week). Select cold-water fatty fish because they have high levels of omega-3 fatty acids.

▲ Use olive oil, peanut oil, or canola oil (all monounsaturated) in limited amounts when you must use fat.

▲ Lose weight if you are overweight. Maintaining a healthy body weight is essential to keeping total cholesterol down, thereby raising HDLs and lowering LDLs.

Finding Your Heart-Risk Ratio

Ideal cholesterol test results should show:

▲ A total cholesterol count of under 200 milligrams

▲ An LDL count that is as low as possible (under 130)

▲ An HDL count that is as high as possible (35 or over)

To determine your heart-risk ratio, divide the total cholesterol count by the HDL count. Ideally, this number should be 4.5, which is the risk ratio, or lower. If, for example your total cholesterol is 180 and your HDL is 40, your heart-risk ratio would be 4.5.

A study at the National Institutes of Health has indicated that for every one percent decrease in blood cholesterol there is a two percent decrease in the chance of coronary artery disease.

If your cholesterol readings indicate you are at risk, it's time to make those dietary changes. Even if you are not at risk today, you'll want to lower the fat and cholesterol in your diet to keep it that way. The chart on the next page shows the cholesterol levels in a variety of foods.

Cholesterol Sources

Food	Amount	Cholesterol (milligrams)
Liver	3.5 oz.	389
Eggs	1 large	213
Shellfish (shrimp)	3 oz., cooked	166
Frankfurter, beef	1 (2 oz.)	35
Frankfurter, turkey	1 frank	39
Veal, roasted	3.5 oz.	103
Leg of lamb, roasted	3.5 oz.	87
Ground beef, broiled	3.5 oz.	101
Chicken breast, roasted	1/2 breast	83
Fish, cod, baked	3 oz.	37
Butter	1 Tbsp.	33
Margarine	1 Tbsp.	0
Whole milk	1 cup	33
Skim milk	1 cup	4
Ice cream, vanilla	1/2 cup	29-45
Ice milk, vanilla	1/2 cup	9
Mozzarella cheese, regular	1 oz.	25
Mozzarella cheese, low-fat	1 oz.	15
Cottage cheese, regular	1/2 cup	17-25
Cottage cheese, low-fat	1/2 cup	10
Yogurt, regular, plain	6 oz.	15
Yogurt, low-fat, plain	6 oz.	0
Yogurt, frozen, chocolate	1/2 cup	3
Doughnut, glazed	1	11

Plant foods such as peanut butter, bread, margarines, shortenings, grains, fruits, and vegetables do not contain cholesterol. Cholesterol is only found in foods of animal origin.

Source: Pennington, J.A.T., Bowes & Church's Food Values of Portions Commonly Used, 16th edition. Philadelphia: J.B. Lippincott, 1994.

Skim the Fat

Chapter 5

How Does Dietary Fat Influence Risk for Disease?

In addition to heart disease and related coronary conditions, research has confirmed that dietary fat plays a critical role in the progression of other diseases as well.

Diet and Cancer

Eating a diet high in fat can increase the risk of developing cancer, particularly cancers of the colon and breast. Studies of cancer rates and eating habits among different world populations show a consistent relationship between high-fat diets and high overall cancer rates. However, none of these population studies is as conclusive as those linking high-fat diets to heart disease.

Several factors appear to play a role in studies of the relationship of dietary fat to the development of cancer, tending to obscure the picture somewhat. High-fat diets tend to be low in complex carbohydrates, fiber, and fruits and vegetables—all thought to help prevent cancer. High-fat diets are also associated with higher intakes of calories and with obesity, both suspected to encourage the development of some cancers.

So it has been difficult to pinpoint connections between dietary fat and specific cancers, or between specific types of fat and cancer. For example, studies of breast cancer support a weak link between dietary fat and the risk of developing breast cancer. Some of the studies also single out saturated fatty acids, but others do not.

What could explain this? For one thing, the amount of fat eaten early in life may have a greater influence on breast cancer risk than fat eaten during adult years. Therefore, when adults lower their fat intake, it might take years to show a beneficial effect on cancer rates.

Another possibility for these somewhat confusing results of population studies is that it is difficult to reconstruct a person's diet over the many years before cancer develops. In addition, population studies are often not sensitive enough to detect links between diet and disease. All this tends to obscure any link between diet and cancer.

But, despite the less-than-conclusive study results, diets high in fat, particularly saturated fatty acids, do appear to increase the risk of developing colon and rectal cancers. There is also evidence of a link between diets high in animal fat and prostate cancer. One study has shown that endometrial cancer occurs more often in parts of the world where the residents eat a high-fat diet. Overall, the evidence is strong enough to support a recommendation to eat less fat in order to reduce the risk of cancer.

The American Cancer Society has made the following recommendations suggesting how nutrition may reduce cancer risk:

▲ *Avoid obesity.*

Studies have found increased rates of cancer of the uterus, kidneys, stomach, colon, and breast in people who are 40 percent or more overweight.

▲ *Cut down on fat intake in order to lower the risk of breast, colon, and prostate cancer.*

The consumption of both saturated fats and unsaturated fats should be reduced in the U.S. diet from the existing average of almost 40 percent to 30 percent or less. Studies show that the amount of fat in the diet can affect the levels of hormones (in particular, prolactin, estrogen, and androgens) which are linked to the development of cancer of the breast and prostate. In colon cancer, studies suggest that high levels of dietary fat cause increased secretion of bile acids into the intestinal tract. Several bile acids have been shown to cause cancer in animals.

▲ *Eat more high fiber foods, such as fruits, vegetables, and whole grain cereals.*

The increased fiber from fruits and vegetables and whole grain cereals and breads speeds the passage of other foods through the intestine, which may reduce the chance for cancer-causing chemicals to have an effect.

▲ *Include foods rich in vitamins A and C in the daily diet.*

Especially important are citrus fruits, which are high in vitamin C, and dark green and deep yellow vegetables, which are high in beta carotene that the body converts into vitamin A. Studies have shown that these two vitamins may help prevent some forms of cancer. But the American Cancer Society strongly warns against supplementing the diet with pill forms of these vitamins, since high doses can have serious side effects. You can get all the vitamins A and C your body can use by choosing at least two helpings daily from the fruit and vegetables mentioned above.

▲ *Include cruciferous vegetables such as cabbage, broccoli, brussels sprouts, kohlrabi, and cauliflower in the diet.*

Evidence from laboratory experiments suggests that some non-nutritive chemicals present in cruciferous vegetables may inhibit the formation of cancer-causing chemicals or reduce cancer incidence in other ways.

▲ *If you drink alcohol, do so in moderation.*

Excessive alcohol consumption has been linked to colon and rectal cancer. The combination of excessive drinking and smoking seems to increase the risk of cancer of the mouth, larynx, esophagus, and respiratory tract.

▲ *Consume moderate amounts of cured and smoked foods.*

Studies of populations in some parts of the world that frequently consume these foods have shown that they have a greater incidence of some cancers, particularly cancer of the stomach and esophagus. Some methods of smoking and pickling foods seem to produce greater amounts of substances called hydrocarbons and nitrosamines, which have been shown to cause cancer in laboratory animals.

Dietary Fat and Hypertension

High blood pressure, discussed in Chapter 3, is a serious health problem in the United States. Uncontrolled hypertension is hazardous to health in many ways. It is the leading cause of stroke and a major contributor to heart and kidney disease.

Although the exact cause of an individual's hypertension is often unknown, various factors are thought to be potential culprits in raising blood pressure:

▲ *High-fat, high-cholesterol diet*

If the arteries become clogged with plaque buildup and fatty deposits, the heart again must work harder to pump blood through them, and the pressure inside the arteries increases as they become more and more clogged. This process can result in hypertension and may be an early sign of coronary heart disease.

▲ *Obesity*

There is a close association between obesity and hypertension. Weight loss decreases blood pressure substantially and often even a loss of 5 to 10 pounds can make a big difference.

▲ *Genetics*

Heredity has a strong influence on an individual's blood pressure. It seems there must be a genetic susceptibility before an individual can develop hypertension. The problem is that most people do not know what their genes have in store for them.

▲ *Stress*

Stressful moments in life can temporarily raise blood pressure. But stress itself does not necessarily lead to hypertension. However, a large amount of psychological stress over many years may contribute to hypertension.

▲ *Tobacco smoking*

Smoking causes a narrowing or tightening of the blood vessels, which causes the heart to work harder to pump blood through them.

▲ *Salt*

Sodium, a major component of table salt, is believed to be the main dietary culprit in hypertension in some people. A high-sodium diet alone, however, does not cause high blood pressure. A combination of factors is involved, including those already discussed here.

▲ *Calcium*

Recent studies have suggested that problems with the body's use of calcium may also be involved in causing hypertension in certain susceptible people. A diet containing adequate amounts of calcium has been shown to lower blood pressure.

▲ *Potassium*

Other studies have pointed to dietary imbalance involving potassium as a factor in the development of hypertension.

▲ *Alcohol*

People who have a high alcohol intake also tend to have high blood pressure.

The National High Blood Pressure Program of the National Heart, Lung, and Blood Institute recommends the following changes in diet and lifestyle to reduce high blood pressure.

▲ *Lose weight.*

Weight reduction should be the first step for people who are more than 10 percent over their desirable weight or have a high percentage of body fat. Weight reduction by caloric restriction often results in a substantial lowering of blood pressure.

▲ *Use alcohol only in moderation.*

If you drink alcohol, curb your consumption. Limit the amount you drink to not more than 1 ounce of alcohol per day (2 ounces of 100 proof liquor, 8 ounces of wine, or 24 ounces of beer).

▲ *Reduce your intake of saturated fats.*

Replace those saturated fats with unsaturated fats and complex carbohydrates.

▲ *Do not smoke.*

▲ *Exercise regularly.*

▲ *Reduce your salt intake if your doctor tells you to.*

A reduced-sodium diet is recommended for some people with a family history of hypertension. If your doctor tells you to follow a low-sodium diet, a registered dietitian can help you plan low-salt meals that taste as good as the salty ones.

Dietary Fat and Diabetes

As we said earlier, there are two types of diabetes: Type I or insulin-dependent diabetes, which occurs suddenly, usually in children or young adults, and Type II, non-insulin dependent, which occurs in adults and often progresses gradually without causing any symptoms. Type II occurs when the body's insulin is no longer effective enough to keep the amount of glucose in the blood at a normal level. The blood glucose level remains consistently elevated in people with Type II diabetes until they are diagnosed and begin treatment.

> Diet is a major factor in Type II diabetes; 80 to 90 percent of the people who develop it are obese.

Actually, obesity can cause the body to become resistant to the action of its own insulin. The pancreas is often producing more than the normal amount of insulin, but the body's cells are resisting the insulin and the blood glucose levels become elevated.

Diet is also a major factor in controlling Type II diabetes. A combination of an individualized meal plan and a regular exercise program will often keep the individual's blood glucose within the normal range. If the person is obese, weight loss often helps control the disease. Sometimes an oral hypoglycemic agent (a pill) or insulin must be used, but the person is usually not dependent on the medication to stay alive, unlike the person with Type I diabetes.

It is important to maintain good control of the blood glucose and blood lipid (fat) levels in both types of diabetes. Consistently high levels can, over the years, cause serious problems such as heart, eye, and kidney disease, nerve damage, and blood circulation problems.

There are strong indications that Type II diabetes can be prevented by good nutrition and maintaining a healthy body weight. For individuals who have a family history of Type II diabetes, it is especially important to make lifestyle changes to prevent the development of the disease. Blood glucose levels should be checked annually, especially after reaching age 30.

The American Diabetes Association has made the following general nutrition recommendations for persons with diabetes:

▲ The emphasis for medical nutrition therapy in Type II diabetes should be placed on achieving glucose, lipid, and blood pressure goals.

▲ A nutritionally adequate meal plan with a reduction of total fat, especially saturated fat, should be employed.

▲ Spacing meals (spreading nutrient intake throughout the day) is another strategy that can be adopted.

▲ Mild to moderate weight loss (10 to 20 pounds) has been shown to improve diabetes control, even if "desirable" body weight is not achieved.

▲ Protein intake should be about 10 to 20 percent of daily calories.

▲ Less than 10 percent of daily calories should be from saturated fats, and dietary cholesterol should be limited to 300 milligrams or less daily.

▲ Daily consumption of a diet containing 20 to 35 grams of dietary fiber from a wide variety of sources is recommended.

▲ For people with mild to moderate hypertension, 2,400 milligrams or less of sodium per day is recommended. For people who have hypertension and kidney disease, 2,000 milligrams or less per day of sodium is recommended.

A recently completed six-month study of adults with Type II diabetes showed significant improvements in blood glucose control when patients received medical nutrition therapy (meal planning and instruction) provided by registered dietitians.

Exactly What is Atherosclerosis?

We've already stated that heart disease is the number one killer in the United States, and the number one cause of heart disease is atherosclerosis, or "hardening of the arteries." Atherosclerosis also contributes to a majority of strokes, the third leading cause of death in the United States.

Atherosclerosis is a condition of adulthood, but it starts when we are children. Lipids, particularly cholesterol and cholesterol linked to fatty acids, begin building up in the muscular walls of the arteries that carry blood throughout the body. The places where lipids accumulate are called fatty streaks.

In adolescence, fatty streaks can grow as more and more cholesterol is incorporated into the arterial walls. The body responds to the presence of fatty streaks by covering them with hard, stiff fibrous tissue and muscle, forming what are called fibrous plaques.

As we move into middle age, the fibrous plaques can continue to grow, accumulating cholesterol, fibrous tissue, and muscle cells. At some point, plaques begin to calcify—that is, calcium deposits form and the plaques harden. The arteries begin to narrow, restricting the flow of blood.

At this stage, several things can happen. The worst (and a relatively common) case is when a stiff, brittle plaque cracks, causing a blood clot to form over the deposit. Often, the additional bulk of the blood clot is enough to block the artery, preventing blood—and the oxygen and nutrients it carries—from reaching tissues downstream from the obstruction. The downstream tissues then die.

> Fortunately, there are indications that the plaque-forming process can be prevented through dietary changes.

The key to atherosclerosis and its reversal lies with the two major carriers of cholesterol—low-density lipoprotein (LDL, the lousy one) and high-density lipo-protein (HDL, the healthy one). LDL particles carry about 60 to 70 percent of the cholesterol moving through the bloodstream, and HDL particles hold between 20 and 30 percent of the total serum cholesterol.

In the simplest terms, too much LDL cholesterol causes cholesterol to accumulate on the walls of blood vessels, leading to fatty streaks, plaques, and blocked arteries.

You may recall that LDL cholesterol and HDL cholesterol have quite different roles in the body. LDL cholesterol delivers cholesterol from the liver to the millions of cells in the body. HDL cholesterol can help to remove cholesterol from the millions of cells in the body and return it to the liver.

In societies in which the population is at a high risk of developing atherosclerosis, such as in the United States, most people have relatively elevated LDL and total cholesterol levels. In addition, the level of HDL cholesterol is an important factor in individual risk.

Lowering the amount of LDL in the blood and raising the amount of HDL can help remove cholesterol from plaques and fatty streaks, preventing further narrowing of arteries. The levels of both LDL and HDL cholesterol in the blood are important factors in assessing risk for heart disease, peripheral artery disease, and stroke.

Peripheral Artery Disease

Muscle damage from atherosclerosis can also happen in the chest, abdomen, legs, and feet. This disorder is known as peripheral artery disease. If the blood supply to the legs or feet is restricted, the result is muscle tiredness and pain upon exertion. When the blood supply to the legs and feet is completely blocked, tissue dies and gangrene results. In the chest and abdominal areas, atherosclerosis can cause the aorta—the main artery—to balloon and rupture, producing life-threatening internal bleeding.

Stroke

When atherosclerosis affects the arteries that supply blood to the brain, a stroke can result. One type of stroke, called a cerebral thrombosis, occurs when a blood clot forms on top of an arterial plaque in a blood vessel in the neck or head. This shuts off or seriously restricts the blood supply to a part of the brain, killing the tissue there in a matter of minutes. This type of stroke typically causes paralysis on one side of the body or disturbances of speech, vision, hearing, or memory.

The exact signs and symptoms of a stroke depend on the specific parts of the brain that are affected. With physical therapy, another part of the brain can sometimes be trained to take over the task once controlled by the damaged area, restoring most or all of the lost functions. A cerebral thrombosis can be fatal, however, if the damage occurs in an area of the brain responsible for breathing.

Atherosclerosis can also cause a second type of stroke—a cerebral hemorrhage—if a plaque-covered artery becomes weak enough to rupture. This happens more frequently in people with high blood pressure, and large parts of the brain can die if the bleeding is severe enough. Cerebral hemorrhage strokes have many of the same symptoms as strokes caused by blood clots, but cerebral hemorrhages are more likely to be fatal.

Skim the Fat

Chapter 6

Building a Lower-Fat Diet

The latest edition of the Dietary Guidelines includes seven practical principles that form the foundation of a healthy diet. In addition to advising people to eat a variety of foods, the guidelines emphasize the importance of choosing foods low in fat, saturated fat, and cholesterol. Recommendations focus on keeping calories from fat to about 30 percent or less of daily total calories. That doesn't mean every single food must be low in fat. You can balance high-fat and low-fat selections over the course of a day or days and still end up within the 30 percent guideline.

Here are the guidelines:

1. Eat a variety of foods.

2. Maintain healthy weight.

3. Choose a diet low in fat, saturated fat, and cholesterol.

4. Choose a diet with plenty of vegetables, fruits, and grain products.

5. Use sugars only in moderation.

6. Use salt and sodium only in moderation.

7. If you drink alcoholic beverages, do so in moderation.

Of course, achieving the right balance requires some knowledge of the fat content of foods. In the USDA's new Food Guide Pyramid, experts break foods into six categories and talk about how to zero in on the leanest selections from each group. The six food groups are

▲ bread, cereal, rice, and pasta

▲ vegetable

▲ fruit

▲ meat, poultry, fish, dry beans, eggs, and nuts

▲ milk, yogurt, and cheese

▲ fats, oils, and sweets

Key

□ FAT (naturally occurring and added)

▼ SUGARS (added)

These symbols show that fat and added sugars come mostly from fats, oils, and sweets but can be part of or added to food from the other food groups as well.

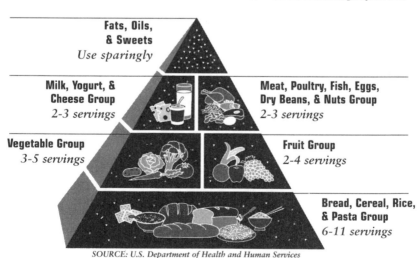

Fats, Oils, & Sweets
Use sparingly

Milk, Yogurt, & Cheese Group
2-3 servings

Meat, Poultry, Fish, Eggs, Dry Beans, & Nuts Group
2-3 servings

Vegetable Group
3-5 servings

Fruit Group
2-4 servings

Bread, Cereal, Rice, & Pasta Group
6-11 servings

SOURCE: *U.S. Department of Health and Human Services*

What's in a Serving?

Here are some serving size examples for each food group. If you eat larger portions, count it as more than one serving. Most Americans are encouraged to eat at least the lowest number of servings from the five food groups each day.

Bread, cereal, rice, and pasta group

— 1 slice of bread

— 1 ounce of ready-to-eat cereal
   (check labels: 1 ounce = 1/4 cup to 2 cups depending on cereal)

— 1/2 cup cooked cereal, rice, or pasta

— 1/2 hamburger roll, bagel, or English muffin

— 3 or 4 plain crackers (small)

Vegetable group

— 1 cup of raw, leafy vegetables

— 1/2 cup of other vegetables, cooked or chopped raw

— 3/4 cup of vegetable juice

Fruit group

— 1 medium apple, banana, orange, nectarine, or peach

— 1/2 cup of chopped, cooked, or canned fruit

— 3/4 cup of fruit juice

Milk, yogurt, and cheese group

— 1 cup of milk or yogurt

— 1 1/2 ounces of natural cheese

— 2 ounces of processed cheese

Meat, poultry, fish, dry beans, eggs, and nuts group

— 2 to 3 ounces of cooked lean meat, poultry, or fish
   (1 ounce of meat = 1/2 cup of cooked dry beans,
   1 egg, or 2 tablespoons of peanut butter)

How Much Should You Eat?

▲ **1200 calories** is the lowest amount recommended to maintain nutritional adequacy. This calorie level is appropriate for weight loss or for extremely inactive individuals.

▲ **1600 calories** is recommended for many sedentary women and some older adults.

▲ **2200 calories** is recommended for most children, teenage girls, active women, and sedentary men. Women who are pregnant or breastfeeding may need more.

▲ **2500 calories** is recommended for teenage boys, active men, and some very active women.

How Big is a Serving Size?

Figuring out the amount of food you should eat is a cinch if you use these images as a guide.

1 ounce of meat	Matchbox
3 ounces of meat	Deck of cards or a bar of soap
8 ounces of meat	Thin paperback book
Medium apple or orange	Tennis ball
Medium potato	Computer mouse
One cup of lettuce	Four green leaves
Slice of bread	Cassette tape
Average bagel	Hockey puck
One ounce of cheese	Four dice
One cup of fruit	Baseball

Bread, Cereal, Rice, and Pasta Group
(Eat 6 to 11 Servings Daily)

It's hard to go wrong emphasizing whole-grain and cereal foods as a big part of a healthy eating style. Health experts encourage Americans to consider grains as the base of a nutritious diet. Not only are oats, wheat, corn, and other grains cholesterol free, but in addition, they carry very little fat. However, some recipes for grain foods can call for the addition of fatty ingredients.

When butter, shortening, oil, or cheese are prominent recipe components, bread products can be quite fatty. Some examples of items on the high-fat list include croissants, Danish pastries, doughnuts, sweet rolls, and cheese breads. For everyday eating, it's best to highlight lower-fat breads, cereals, and whole grains.

Choose Lower-Fat Grain Items More Often

▲ sandwich breads, such as wheat, rye, white

▲ English muffins

▲ hot dog and hamburger buns

▲ bagels

▲ pita or pocket bread

▲ unfried tortillas (corn, flour)

▲ plain pasta, noodles, rice

▲ oatmeal, grits, farina

▲ dry cereals, except regular granola

▲ crackers, such as graham crackers, matzos, saltines, melba toast, flatbreads, breadsticks

▲ pretzels, air-popped popcorn

▲ fig and low-fat fruit bars, gingersnaps, vanilla wafers, animal crackers

Choose Higher-Fat Grain Items Less Often

▲ butter rolls

▲ cheese breads, croissants

▲ doughnuts

▲ oversized muffins

▲ biscuits

▲ convenience pasta mixes with cheese or cream sauces

▲ fried rice

▲ regular granola

▲ corn chips, potato chips, pork rinds

▲ butter-flavored and cheese-flavored crackers

▲ chocolate chip and bakery cookies, frosted cookies

▲ bagel chips

If you want a more specific picture of the fat content of various bread and grain products, the following list should help. And remember, consult the Nutrition Facts available on most products.

Fat Content of Bread, Cereal, Rice, and Pasta

Item	Serving Size	Grams of Fat
Rice, pasta, cooked,	1/2 cup	Trace
Bread	1 slice	1
Hamburger roll, bagel	1	2
English muffin	1	2
Tortilla	8-inch diameter	3
Crackers plain	small, 3-4	3
Pancakes	4-inch diameter, 2	3
Cookies plain	medium, 2	4
Doughnut, medium	1	11
Croissant	large	12
Danish	medium	13
Cake, frosted	medium, 1/16	13
Pie, fruit	8-inch diameter, 1/6	19

Adapted from USDA's Food Guide Pyramid. US Department of Agriculture, Human Nutrition Information Service; April 1992. Home and Garden Bulletin 249.

Vegetable Group
(Eat 3 to 5 Servings Daily)

Vegetables are naturally low in fat and contain no cholesterol. The only way to sabotage their heart-healthy profile is to load butter, margarine, rich cream sauces, or large quantities of cheese onto them during cooking.

Frozen or convenience vegetable products can be the biggest offenders. Many come already cooked with extra fats. A better alternative to heating frozen broccoli with cheese sauce might be to take plain frozen broccoli, cook it, and then add a squeeze of lemon and a sprinkle of Parmesan cheese.

Fat Content of Various Vegetables

Item	Serving Size	Grams of Fat
Vegetables, cooked	1/2 cup	Trace
Vegetables, leafy, raw	1 cup	Trace
Vegetables, nonleafy, raw	1/2 cup	Trace
Potatoes, scalloped	1/2 cup	4
Potato salad	1/2 cup	8
French fries	10	8

Adapted from USDA's Food Guide Pyramid. US Department of Agriculture, Human Nutrition Information Service; April 1992. Home and Garden Bulletin 249.

Choose Lower-Fat Vegetable Items More Often

▲ fresh vegetables

▲ frozen vegetables without sauce or butter

▲ canned vegetables without sauce or butter

Choose Higher-Fat Vegetable Items Less Often

▲ frozen vegetables with cheese, cream, or butter sauce

▲ asparagus with hollandaise sauce

▲ french fries

▲ scalloped potatoes

▲ potato salad

▲ fried zucchini, eggplant Parmesan

When You Can't Measure. . .

When you're in a situation where you can't measure out your vegetables, how do you know when you have a 1/2-cup serving? Because there is no one way to visualize a half cup, we came up with the following specific amounts:

▲ 6 asparagus spears

▲ 7 or 8 baby carrots or carrot sticks

▲ 1 ear of corn on the cob

▲ 3 to 5 spears of broccoli

Each of these amounts is equivalent to a 1/2-cup serving.

Fruit Group
(Eat 2 to 4 Servings Daily)

Like vegetables, most fruits are low in fat and cholesterol free. Two exceptions are coconut and avocado. Coconut is high in total fat and high in saturated fat, the type of fat that can raise blood cholesterol levels. The bulk of the fat found in an avocado, on the other hand, is monounsaturated.

Any kind of fresh or frozen fruit or juice fits easily into a low-fat diet. Of course, whole fresh fruits (apples with skin, pears, plums) have more fiber than frozen juices, or canned fruits. Some of that fiber may help lower blood cholesterol levels. An example is the soluble fiber pectin, which is found in apples.

Choose Lower-Fat Fruits More Often

▲ fresh fruits, except avocados and coconuts

▲ dried fruits, such as raisins and prunes

▲ canned fruits

▲ frozen fruits

Choose Higher-Fat Fruits Less Often

▲ avocados, guacamole

▲ coconuts, coconut milk

A list of the fat content of different fruits is on the next page. It's easy to see that fruits, with two minor exceptions, are low-fat foods.

Fat Content of Various Fruits		
Item	Serving Size	Grams of Fat
Whole fruit: apple, orange	1 medium	Trace
Fruit, raw or canned	1/2 cup	Trace
Fruit juice, unsweetened	3/4 cup	Trace
Avocado	1/4	9
Coconut, dried	1/3 cup	9

Adapted from USDA's Food Guide Pyramid. US Department of Agriculture, Human Nutrition Information Service; April 1992. Home and Garden Bulletin 249

Milk, Yogurt, and Cheese Group (Eat 2 to 3 Servings Daily)

Some daily foods contain cholesterol as well as larger amounts of fat and saturated fat, so you'll need to be more judicious when choosing foods from this group. Whole milk, for instance, carries about 8 grams of fat per cup. To decrease high fat totals, gradually wean yourself away from whole-milk dairy foods to products made with skim or low-fat milk. If the thought of drinking skim milk turns you off, consider mixing whole milk with 2%, then mix 2% with 1%, and so on, until you have adjusted to the taste of skim.

Start using skim milk in recipes for pudding, sauce, soup, and bakery products. Skim or low-fat milk is also an excellent "creamer" for coffee, much more healthful than nondairy creamers, which are low in cholesterol but high in fat. Chances are you won't be able to tell the difference. Moreover, the calcium content of low-fat dairy products is equivalent to full-fat

Fat Content of Milk, Yogurt, and Cheese

Item	Serving Size	Grams of Fat
Skim milk	1 cup	Trace
1% milk	1 cup	2.6
2% milk	1 cup	5
2% milk, chocolate	1 cup	5
Whole milk	1 cup	8
Nonfat yogurt, plain	8 ounces	Trace
Low-fat yogurt, fruit	8 ounces	3
Low-fat yogurt, plain	8 ounces	4
Cottage cheese, 4% fat	1/2 cup	5
Mozzarella part skim, grated	1/2 cup	7
Ricotta, part skim	1/2 cup	10
Cheddar cheese, natural	1 1/2 ounces	14
Cheese, processed	2 ounces	18
Frozen yogurt	1/2 cup	2
Ice milk	1/2 cup	3
Ice cream	1/2 cup	7
Premium ice cream	1/2 cup	14

Adapted from USDA's Food Guide Pyramid. US Department of Agriculture, Human Nutrition Information Service; April 1992. Home and Garden Bulletin 249

dairy foods, so you won't be losing out on this bone-strengthening mineral.

Lower-fat cheeses are another way to trim fat in the diet. Many hard cheeses carry 10 or more grams of fat in a 1-ounce portion. Reduced fat selections carry one-third to one-half that amount. However, when fat is removed from cheese, both the flavor and texture can be altered. Some manufacturers are making fat-free cheeses available. The best strategy is to try a variety of lower-fat options and find the ones that are acceptable to your taste buds.

Choose Lower-Fat Dairy Products More Often

- ▲ skim milk
- ▲ 1% milk
- ▲ buttermilk made from skim milk
- ▲ evaporated skim milk
- ▲ nonfat milk powder
- ▲ 1%, low-fat, or fat-free cottage cheese
- ▲ low-fat or fat-free ice cream
- ▲ nonfat and low-fat yogurts
- ▲ reduced-fat or fat-free sour cream
- ▲ nonfat cream cheese
- ▲ nonfat or low-fat cheese

Choose Higher-Fat Dairy Products Less Often

- ▲ whole milk
- ▲ evaporated milk
- ▲ sweetened condensed milk
- ▲ buttermilk made from whole milk
- ▲ creamed cottage cheese (4% fat)
- ▲ cream cheese
- ▲ hard cheeses, such as cheddar and Swiss

▲ processed cheese spreads and dips

▲ ice cream (particularly premium)

▲ sour cream

▲ whipped cream

▲ half-and-half

The list on page 58 gives you an idea of the number of grams of fat in various dairy foods. Remember, you can read the nutrition label for more details on specific brands of dairy foods.

Meat, Poultry, Fish, Dry Beans, Eggs, and Nuts Group (Eat 5 to 7 Ounces Daily)

The meat group is an excellent place to start trimming the fat in your diet. Although it's easier nowadays to find meats trimmed of most of their fat, and chicken is often sold without the skin, health experts feel there is plenty of room for improvement when it comes to reducing fat from meat.

Notice, the idea is to cut down on meat, not eliminate it completely. Contrary to popular belief, red meat need not be totally avoided, especially since it is a good source of iron, zinc, and several other important nutrients, nutrients somewhat difficult to find in adequate amounts in other foods.

The smart approach to red meat is to search out leaner cuts, such as beef round, rump, and sirloin tip. When buying pork, look for the tenderloin and loin cuts. Leg of lamb is leaner than lamb chops, and practically all cuts of veal are low in fat but rather high in cholesterol. It's pretty hard to go wrong with chicken, although the dark meat does have a bit more fat than the light meat.

Fish is naturally low in saturated fat. Some of the fattier varieties, such as salmon, mackerel, and bluefish, contain high levels of omega-3 polyunsaturated fats. Studies suggest that foods rich in omega-3 fatty acids may be helpful in warding off heart disease.

Richest sources of omega-3 include mackerel, anchovies, herring, salmon, sardines, lake trout, Atlantic sturgeon, and fresh tuna. Moderate amounts are found in turbot, bluefish, striped bass, shark, rainbow smelt, swordfish, and rainbow trout. Shellfish—crab, lobster, shrimp, mussels, oysters, clams, and squid—contain lesser amounts.

Studies show that eating an ounce of fish a day, or a couple of servings 2 or 3 times per week, slashes your chances of heart attack by one-third to one-half.

Another way to trim the fat is to use meat substitutes, like dry beans and peas, which are nearly as high in protein as meat but

Fat Content of Meat, Meat Substitutes

Item	Serving Size	Grams of Fat
Lean meat, poultry, fish, cooked	3 ounces	6
Chicken, with skin, fried	3 ounces	13
Ground beef, lean, cooked	3 ounces	16
Bologna	1 ounce	16
Dry beans, peas, cooked	1/2 cup*	Trace
Egg	1*	5
Peanut butter	2 tablespoons*	15
Nuts	1/3 cup or 1 ounce	22

*Count 1 egg, 1/2 cup dry beans and peas, or 2 tablespoons peanut butter as 1 ounce of meat.

Adapted from USDA's Food Guide Pyramid. US Department of Agriculture, Human Nutrition Information Service; April 1992. Home and Garden Bulletin 249

much lower in fat. Combined with rice or other grains, legumes like kidney beans or black-eyed peas make high-quality meat replacements.

Choose Leaner Meat or Meat Replacements More Often

▲ chicken, turkey (remove the skin)

▲ eye of the round, round steak

▲ extra-lean ground sirloin

▲ veal

▲ pork loin and tenderloin

▲ wild game, such as rabbit, pheasant, venison

▲ tuna canned in water

▲ cod, haddock, pollack

▲ dry beans, split peas

▲ egg whites

▲ lean lunch meat like turkey, chicken breast, ham

Choose Higher-Fat Meat Items Less Often

▲ goose, domestic duck

▲ prime beef, heavily marbled meats

▲ corned beef, pastrami

▲ spareribs, rib eye roast, steak

▲ regular ground meat

▲ hot dogs, sausage, bologna

▲ bacon

▲ liverwurst

▲ refried beans cooked with lard
(check the label for fat content)

Fats, Oils, and Sweets Group (Use Sparingly)

A low-fat style of eating allows room for the use of some fats and higher-fat foods. Remember, the whole idea of low-fat eating is to balance low-fat and high-fat selections. The sixth food group of the USDA Food Guide Pyramid singles out added fats—butter, margarine, salad dressing—and encourages Americans to use these items sparingly. Because many people

Fat Content of Fats, Oils, and Sweets

Item	Serving Size	Grams of Fat
Butter, margarine	1 tablespoon	12
Mayonnaise	1 tablespoon	11
Low-fat mayonnaise	1 tablespoon	5
Sour cream	1 tablespoon	3
Lite sour cream	1 tablespoon	0.7
Salad dressing	1 tablespoon	7
Low-fat salad dressing	1 tablespoon	4
Cream cheese	1 ounce	10
Frozen yogurt	1/2 cup	2
Fruit sorbet	1/2 cup	0
Gelatin dessert	1/2 cup	0
Sherbet	1/2 cup	2
Chocolate bar	1 ounce	9

Adapted from USDA's Food Guide Pyramid. US Department of Agriculture, Human Nutrition Information Service; April 1992. Home and Garden Bulletin 249

overdo it with foods from this category, it would pay to become more familiar with the fat content of these items.

Salt

In addition to the guidelines from the Food Pyramid, the Dietary Guidelines for Americans include advice about using salt and sodium in moderation. Here's some additional information with advice for what to use instead of salt to enhance food flavors.

Salt is the leading additive in many processed foods and often is added at the dining table. But the truth is that there is enough sodium naturally present in the foods we eat and in our water supply to more than meet our daily needs.

Common words for sodium

Watch food labels for sources of sodium, which may be listed as:

salt • sodium • brine • broth • cured • corned
pickled • smoked • soy sauce • teriyaki sauce
monosodium glutamate (MSG)
sodium bicarbonate (baking soda) • sodium aluminum sulfate
(baking powder) • disodium phosphate • sodium benzoate

What to use in place of salt

Certain foods are known for their high sodium content—snack foods (such as salted chips, salted crackers and nuts, condiments, and cured and processed meats); canned foods (such as vegetables, beans, and fish); cheeses; and boxed convenience foods (such as macaroni and cheese, pasta mixes, or rice side dishes). Fresh foods are an ideal choice when you are trying to reduce sodium, but processed foods can be a part of your eating plan, too. With a little creativity, high-sodium foods can be replaced with flavorful low-sodium substitutes. The switch will open up a whole new world of tastes.

To Lower Your Salt Intake

Choose less often:

1/2 cup canned tuna (310 mg. sodium)

1 medium dill pickle (418 mg. sodium)

3 ounces of ham (1100 mg. sodium)

3 cups of regular microwave popcorn (190 mg. sodium)

1 cup of boxed convenience rice side dish (1560 mg. sodium)

1 cup of chicken vegetable soup (1068 mg. sodium)

1/2 cup canned green beans (170 mg. sodium)

Choose more often:

1/2 cup low-sodium canned tuna (79 mg. sodium)

1 medium cucumber marinated in vinegar (5 mg. sodium)

3 ounces of lean pork loin (64 mg. sodium)

3 cups of air-popped popcorn (0 sodium) OR 3 cups of salt-free microwave popcorn (0 sodium)

1 cup of plain brown or white rice seasoned with herbs (9 mg. sodium)

1 cup of low-sodium chicken vegetable soup (90 mg. sodium)

1/2 cup fresh green beans (2 mg. sodium) OR 1/2 cup frozen green beans (3 mg. sodium) OR 1/2 cup canned no-salt-added green beans (1 mg. sodium)

Skim the Fat

Chapter 7

Fat Fighting Made Simple

If the concept of setting a fat budget has you confused, take heart. There is a simple way to start cutting fat out of your diet. Use these six shortcut steps to build a more healthful, leaner style of eating.

1

Double up on grains, vegetables, and fruits at mealtime. Fill up two-thirds of your meal plate with these foods to help shift the focus away from higher-fat animal foods.

Doubling up on grains, vegetables, and fruits at mealtime can be easy, especially if you become familiar with the many virtues of these foods. Choose whole grain, unrefined carbohydrates more often. These include whole grain breads, cereals, and pastas, as well as legumes, potatoes, and corn. All are all low in fat but high in vitamins, minerals, and fiber.

Choose these:

▲ Whole wheat flour

▲ Brown rice, wild rice, pilaf mix, or any other whole grain rice

▲ Bulgur, barley

▲ Oat bran, oatmeal

▲ Whole grain cereals without sugar added, such as wheat and bran, oatmeal, and oat bran flakes.

▲ Whole grain breads without sugar added, such as whole wheat, rye, pumpernickel, sourdough, whole wheat pita bread, tortillas, or bagels

▲ Homemade muffins, pancakes, waffles, and cornbread

▲ Air-popped popcorn, whole wheat pretzels without added shortening

▲ Rye or whole wheat melba toast, rye crackers, flatbread, matzo crackers, whole wheat bread sticks, or brown rice crackers

Pasta

▲ All types, including whole wheat or any pasta made from whole-grain or semolina flour

▲ Suggested sauces include marinara with no meat added, fresh tomato and basil, primavera, or red clam

Beans and Legumes

▲ All dried or canned beans, lentils, and the like

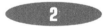

Practice the less-is-more approach to meat. Trim portions to a moderate 2 or 3 ounces. (Three ounces is about the size of a deck of cards.) Try mixing meats into a stir-fry or casserole at first to help take the focus off smaller portions.

When practicing this less-is-more approach to meats, remember that portion control is critical. Try to limit meats to 6 ounces or less per day. A skinless chicken breast or a piece of meat about the size of a deck of cards weighs about 3 ounces.

Using that same amount of chicken breast as part of a stir-fry dish mixed with lots of colorful, crisp vegetables, served over rice, makes it go a lot further. Fill your plate with the grains and vegetables, and you'll still enjoy your meat and poultry but in smaller (healthier) portions.

3

Wean yourself away from whole milk and high-fat dairy products. You get just as much calcium from skim and 1% milk products, with much less fat.

If you need more calcium than you are getting (and remember that around menopause, women need about 1500 milligrams a day), check with your dietitian for a more comprehensive list of foods that are rich in calcium.

Sources of Calcium				
Food	Amount	Calories	Fat	Calcium
Milk				
Skim	8 oz.	86	0.5 gm.	302 mg.
1%	8 oz.	103	2.6 gm.	313 mg.
2%	8 oz.	121	4.7 gm.	297 mg.
Whole	8 oz.	150	8.2 gm.	291 mg.
Yogurt				
Whole	8 oz.	144	7.4 gm.	274 mg.
Low-fat	8 oz.	139	4 gm.	400 mg.
Ice Cream				
Regular	1/2 cup	132	7.3 gm.	87 mg.
Premium	1/2 cup	178	12 gm.	78 mg.
Ice Milk				
Vanilla	1/2 cup	92	2.8 gm.	92 mg.
Cheese				
Swiss	1 oz.	95	7.1 gm.	219 mg.
American	1 oz.	106	8.9 gm.	124 mg.
Mozzarella	1 oz.	80	6.1 gm.	105 mg.
Mozzarella, part skim	1 oz.	72	4.5 gm.	131 mg.
Cottage cheese				
Low-fat (1%)	1 cup	164	2.3 gm.	138 mg.
Low-fat (2%)	1 cup	203	4.4 gm.	155 mg.
Creamed (4%)	1 cup	217	9.5 mg.	126 mg.

Source: Pennington, J.A.T., Bowes & Church's Food Values of Portions Commonly Used, 16th ed. Philadelphia, J.B. Lippincott, 1994.

Skim the Fat

Cook with less fat. Steam, microwave, stir-fry, roast, or grill foods. Add citrus juices, wine, and herbs for flavor instead of fat. Use vegetable cooking spray to replace margarine or oil.

When you cook meat, use the leaner cuts and follow these tips for cooking:

▲ Do not overcook. Keep the meats moist by slow cooking.

▲ Use slow, moist cooking methods like braising and stewing for maximum flavor and tenderness.

▲ To prevent natural juices from escaping, avoid pricking or searing steaks while cooking.

▲ Don't salt the meat before you cook it. Salting beforehand tends to delay browning and draws out moisture.

▲ Marinate meats overnight when possible to increase tenderness. Marinades that include an acid ingredient, like wine, vinegar, or lemon juice, will help break down some of the protein, making the meat even more tender.

With beef, try grilling, broiling, roasting, or simmering in wine or broth. Also, remember that 3 ounces of cooked beef (that's about 4 ounces raw) is a healthful portion at one sitting. That serving size is roughly the size of a deck of cards or the palm of your hand. If that seems like too little, remember, you only need a little protein. So a little bit will do you just fine. Other protein choices, in 3-ounce cooked portions, include:

▲ Pork tenderloin with 142 calories, 4.1 gm. fat

▲ Leg shank portion of lamb with 193 calories, 10.7 gm. fat.

▲ Sirloin portion of leg of lamb with 250 calories, 17 gm. fat.

▲ Skinless chicken breast with 163 calories, 6.3 gm. fat.

▲ Skinless turkey breast with 95 calories, 3.2 gm. fat.

Calorie and fat content of the leanest cuts of beef

Per 3 ounces, cooked, trimmed of all fat	Calories	Grams of fat
Top round (London broil)	162 calories	5.4 gm.
Eye of the round	156 calories	5.4 gm.
Round tip, sirloin tip	162 calories	6.3 gm.
Top sirloin steak	177 calories	7.5 gm.
Tenderloin	174 calories	8.1 gm.

Source: Pennington, J.A.T., Bowes & Church's Food Values of Portions Commonly Used, 16th ed. Philadelphia, J.B. Lippincott, 1994.

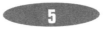

Read labels of snacks and precooked convenience foods you buy. If you are having trouble identifying low-fat choices, use the 3-gram rule. If a product has 3 grams of fat or less per 100-calorie serving, it falls within recommended fat guidelines.

If you want snacks, make them low-fat and healthful by following the tips below:

▲ Keep sliced fruit, as well as whole fresh fruit, available.

▲ Keep prepared, raw vegetables available for munching.

▲ Keep a variety of low-fat breads and muffins on hand.

▲ Snack on low-sugar cereals, either dry or with nonfat milk.

▲ Snack on plain, low-fat yogurt with fruit, cereal, or bread.

▲ Freeze fruit juice to use as snacks on hot days.

Snacking can actually be helpful in fighting fat, especially if a snack takes the edge off hunger that could otherwise lead to overeating. Here are some ideas for choosing your snacks.

Lower-Fat Snacks	
Choose more often:	**Choose less often:**
Baked tortilla chips	Corn chips
Pretzels	Potato chips
Bagel with fat-free	
cheese or fruit	Doughnut
Spiced applesauce	Apple pie
Nonfat frozen yogurt	Ice cream
Low-fat string cheese	Cheddar cheese
Soft pretzel	Croissant
Fruit smoothie	
or nonfat yogurt shake	Milk shake
Salsa	Sour cream-based dip
Frozen juice bar	Ice cream bar
Angel food cake	Pound cake

Practice the art of fat balancing. You don't have to be a math wizard to know that premium ice cream, potato chips, and football-size burgers are high in fat. Try eating these foods less frequently and in smaller amounts. If you do have a meal high in fat, be sure the next one is low to keep your day in balance.

Meticulously tracking your food and fat calories at every meal is unrealistic. But you can learn enough food values for typical meals to help you estimate how you're doing. Remember, one sure way to curb the fat in any meal is to consume most of it as grains, vegetables, or fruits.

44 Fat-Trimming Tips

Bringing fat levels into line with health recommendations is not as difficult as most people seem to think. It's a simple goal, easily accomplished by shaving a few grams of fat here and a few grams of fat there. These 44 suggestions offer help to get you started.

Meat Fat Savings

1

Take the focus off small meat portions by trying stir-frys. Very little or no oil and lots of vegetables keep the dish lean.

2

Try the en papillote (paper packet) technique for fish or chicken. Use parchment paper or foil and place lean meat, herbs, vegetables, and a splash of liquid, like wine, in the center. Wrap and bake.

3

Bake fish with a splash of white wine, chopped tomatoes, and basil for a fast, low-fat entree.

4

Opt for the "select" grade in meat; it has less marbling (and so, much less fat) than choice cuts.

5

Marinate lean cuts of meats with citrus juice, vinegar, or other acidic liquids to help tenderize them before cooking. Add fresh herbs to flavor marinade.

6

Substitute turkey breast or lean ham for luncheon meats like bologna, salami, and liverwurst. Or try low-fat turkey copycat versions of pastrami and bologna.

7

Let lean smoked ham or Canadian bacon take the place of bacon in recipes. Ham offers bacon's smoky flavor with less fat.

8

Use meat and cheese as side dishes, and let vegetables and grains fill out the plate.

9

Peel the skin off chicken or turkey after roasting or baking. As long as you remove skin prior to eating, you'll cut back on fat.

10

Broil meats used in stews, soups, and roasts rather than browning them in oil. No need to add more fat to foods that already contain plenty.

11

Oven-fry chicken and fish: dip in egg whites, coat with seasoned bread crumbs, and bake on a nonstick pan coated with vegetable spray.

Leaning Toward Desserts

12

Make fruit pies with a single crust. Place the fruit directly in the pie dish and top with pastry. Or make an open-face fruit tart.

13

Bake, stew, or poach peaches (or apples or pears) with cinnamon, cloves, and honey for a lean dessert splurge.

14

Puree chopped cantaloupe in the blender; add a dash of nutmeg, and serve the sauce over ice milk or low-fat frozen yogurt.

15

Substitute evaporated skim milk in recipes that call for heavy cream.

16

Reach for gingersnaps, vanilla wafers, graham crackers, fig or low-fat fruit bars, and animal crackers when cookie cravings strike.

17

Serve angel food cake with fresh strawberries (or frozen, thawed with syrup included) and fresh kiwi slices for a colorful dessert.

18

Make pudding with skim milk. Add a touch of spice, like nutmeg, cinnamon, or cloves, to boost flavor.

Vegetable Cookery

19

Cook onions, mushrooms, and green peppers in a pan coated with nonstick vegetable spray, not oil. Two tablespoons of oil used to saute vegetables will carry an extra 240 fat calories; vegetable sprays add less than 10.

20

Cut back on buttering vegetables with this gradual method: use one part margarine with one part lemon juice. Eventually try for mostly lemon and little or no margarine.

21

Top a baked potato with salsa, meatless chili, or low-fat cottage cheese and dill or mixed vegetables plus a tablespoon of grated low-fat cheese.

22

Roast vegetables (sweet pepper chunks, zucchini, asparagus, sliced eggplant) for some low-fat flavor. Spray lightly with vegetable spray; bake for about 15 minutes at 400°F or until tender but crisp.

23

Peel and chop jicama or cucumbers; sprinkle with chili powder to make a Tex-Mex-style munchie.

Sauces, Condiments

24

Create a tangy salad dressing with a splash of rice vinegar and dried herbs, or combine plain nonfat yogurt, Dijon mustard, and spices for a creamier topping.

25

Fix a mock cream sauce with nonfat, plain yogurt; season with dill and serve over salmon. Another variation: season yogurt with horseradish and serve warm instead of chilled.

26

Save roughly 10 grams of fat by substituting a tablespoon of mustard for a tablespoon of mayonnaise on a sandwich. Other low-fat spreads include fruit and vegetable chutney and salsa.

27

Substitute low-fat milk and chicken stock for cream in recipes. The flavor will be less rich, but will taste as good.

28

Keep reduced-fat margarines and mayonnaise on hand; they often contain half the fat of the full-fat variety. Nonfat mayonnaise is another option.

29

Use nonfat powdered milk to lighten coffee instead of cream or nondairy creamers.

30

Pour syrup on pancakes or waffles instead of butter. Two tablespoons contain 100 calories, but zero fat. Two tablespoons of butter add 200 calories, almost all from fat.

31

Revamp vinaigrette dressing recipes from traditional 3 part oil, 1 part vinegar to 3 parts vinegar, 1 part oil. Use rice vinegar for a milder flavor.

32

Mix equal amounts of nonfat plain yogurt with mayonnaise to make a creamy, lower-fat dressing for tuna or chicken salad. For even more savings, use reduced-fat or fat-free mayonnaise.

General Strategies

33

Concentrate on a few target foods that you're willing to substitute for or limit. Starting with small changes allows for a better long-term adjustment to low-fat eating.

34

Look for crackers and snack products that have been baked rather than fried. Be sure to read the Nutrition Facts panel.

35

Chill homemade and canned soups; skim off the fat layer that forms on the top. Each tablespoon discarded saves about 120 fat calories.

36

Let an 8-ounce container of 99 percent fat-free cottage cheese stand in for the ricotta cheese in your lasagna recipe. You save almost 200 calories, most of them from fat. Nonfat and low-fat ricotta cheeses are also available.

37

Order pizza with any kind of vegetables—onions, broccoli, mushrooms, green pepper—and less cheese. For a meat topping, choose Canadian bacon or ham instead of high-fat items like pepperoni and sausage.

38

Drain pan-fried foods on a paper towel before serving to absorb extra grease. Go easy on the oil.

39

Keep the oil in your saucepan or wok very hot when stir-frying. Vegetables soak up cold oil much quicker than hot.

40

Sprinkle powdered butter substitutes (found in the spice section) onto hot foods like baked squash and mashed potatoes. One half teaspoon, a mere 4 calories, replaces the 108 calories and 12 grams of fat found in a tablespoon of butter.

41

Fill the refrigerator with nonfat yogurts, sliced raw veggies, seasonal fresh fruits, fruit juice bars, and frozen low-fat fudge bars. When the urge to snack strikes, these low-fat munchies will be at your fingertips.

42

Nibble on breadsticks instead of buttery dinner or crescent rolls. Breadsticks are much lower in fat, and there is less temptation to slather them with butter.

43

Experiment with fresh herbs like basil, dill, rosemary, and cilantro. Try them on vegetables and poultry and in soups. They add lots of great flavor but no fat.

44

Give yourself a break on occasion. When you're tired of paying attention to every bite of food you put into your mouth and craving a few french fries or a slice of chocolate cake, indulge and enjoy yourself! For heart and overall health, diets don't have to include only certain foods. It bears repeating: Low fat eating is all a matter of balance.

Stocking the Lower-Fat Kitchen

Here's a list of healthful foods you may want to have on hand for your new low-fat lifestyle:

In the Fridge

Nonfat or skim milk—Use with whole grain cereals, in cooking and baking, or just to drink.

Nonfat plain or fruit yogurt—Use in salad dressings, cooking, or as a food itself.

Tofu—Use in stir-frys, salad dressings, and sauces.

Part-skim ricotta cheese—Use sparingly as a spread on bread or in limited amounts in cooking.

1%-fat cottage cheese—Use in limited amounts when recipes call for cream cheese.

Part-skim mozzarella cheese—Use in limited amounts in cooking.

Low-calorie Italian or vinaigrette salad dressings—The calorie count should be no more than 10 calories per tablespoon. Check the sodium content, however, because often in lowering calories, excess salt is added for flavor.

Reduced calorie, no-cholesterol mayonnaise—Use sparingly, as it does contain fat calories.

Olive oil—A little goes a long way, and it's believed to raise your HDL cholesterol (that's the healthy one).

Safflower oil, sunflower oil, or canola oil—Canola oil, made from rapeseed, has the lowest amount of saturated fat of any oil. Keep oils refrigerated.

Extra-large eggs—Use only the whites, so these are the best buy.

Egg substitute (low-fat, cholesterol-free)—for use when eggs can be eliminated altogether.

Chopped or crushed garlic—a readily available seasoning for many foods. It loses flavor in storage, however.

All-fruit preserves—a good substitute spread for butter or margarine.

Fruits—Use seasonal fresh fruit preferably, particularly apples, pears, oranges, and grapefruit, because they are higher in the fiber that lowers cholesterol. If fresh is not available, use frozen unsweetened fruit and fruit juice concentrate, canned fruit without sugar added, or dried fruit. Have lemons on hand as a seasoning for salads and on seafood.

Vegetables—Whenever possible, use fresh seasonal vegetables; their flavor is best. However, for convenience, frozen or canned (without sauces) work well. Salad greens, green and red peppers, carrots, tomatoes, broccoli, cauliflower, and cucumbers are particularly good because they are high in fiber, which aids digestion. Prepare by steaming or microwaving.

In the Pantry

Choose whole grain, unrefined carbohydrates such as whole grain breads, cereals, and pastas, as well as legumes, potatoes, and corn. They are all low in fat but high in vitamins, minerals, and fiber.

Canned goods that have added fat or meat or high sodium levels should be avoided. Select salt-reduced products if salt-free are not available. Rinse salted canned products to remove added salt.

Nonstick cooking spray—Use in cooking instead of butter or oil.

Powdered butter substitutes—Use to season vegetables or popcorn.

Dried split peas, beans, and lentils—These are high in fiber.

Brown rice, wild rice, barley, bulgur, pilaf mix, and other whole grains—These are also high in fiber. (If brown rice is kept a long time, store it in the refrigerator or freezer to keep it from becoming rancid.)

Pasta—Try whole-grain pastas or those made with semolina and no egg yolks. Try quinoa pasta for variety.

Oat bran—This is a great source of fiber. Use as a hot cereal or in baking and cooking whenever possible. Store in refrigerator or freezer.

Oatmeal, steel-cut oats, oat bran cereal—All these cereals are high in fiber.

Shredded wheat-style biscuits with added bran—This salt-free, sugar-free, whole-grain cereal high in insoluble fiber.

Canned Goods

Salmon (pink or red)—high in omega-3 fatty acids

Albacore tuna in water—contains omega-3 fatty acids

Unsweetened fruit in natural juice

Whole-kernel corn (preferably sodium-reduced)—high in fiber

Kidney, pinto, and garbanzo beans—high in fiber

Black-eyed peas—high in fiber

Sodium-reduced chicken broth, defatted

Sodium-reduced or salt-free tomato paste, tomato sauce, dried tomatoes, and Italian plum tomatoes

Sodium-reduced or salt-free marinara sauce (no meat added)

Vegetarian split-pea soup or lentil soup—high in fiber

Sodium-reduced vegetable juice

Seasonings

Balsamic, red, or white wine,
and brown rice vinegars

Sodium-reduced soy sauce

Dijon mustard

Worcestershire sauce
(use in limited amounts)

Salt-free vegetable seasonings

Fresh garlic

Garlic and onion powders (not salts)

Italian herb blend

Crushed red pepper flakes

Dried thyme, dill, bay leaves, and any other of your
favorite herbs and spices

Black peppercorns (in mill for fresh grinding)

Dehydrated onion, garlic, shallot,
and vegetable flakes

Hungarian paprika (once opened,
store in refrigerator)

Nutmeg (preferably whole,
to be used with grater)

Ground cinnamon

Pure vanilla extract

Dairy Products

Nonfat evaporated milk—also called evaporated skim milk. Use for cooking and baking.

Nonfat powdered milk—also called dried skim milk. Use as a lightener in coffee instead of most nondairy creamers that may be high in tropical oils and/or saturated fats.

Snacks

Brown rice **crackers**, whole wheat matzo wafers, or other crackers that are whole grain **with no fat added**. Pretzels and fat-free tortilla chips are also good choices.

Popcorn—low-calorie, high fiber. Make in an air popper or microwave. Make sure no butter or oil has been added. Read the nutrition facts panel for sodium content.

For the Freezer

The freezer offers an emergency supply of items that can help you put together healthful meals without running to the grocery store. While fresh fruits and vegetables in season have wonderful flavor, foods properly frozen and stored still have good flavor and food value, and they are convenient.

Frozen vegetables—particularly corn, peas, and mixed beans, which are high in fiber and can be added to salads as well as served as vegetables. Avoid any vegetables frozen in butter or other sauces.

Frozen pasta and vegetable mix—Use as a salad, hot side dish, or stir-fried.

Natural fruit juice bars—an acceptable sweet snack.

Frozen unsweetened fruit juice concentrates—apple, pear, grape, pineapple, or orange, all to be used in cooking.

Unsweetened frozen fruit

Freshly grated Reggiano Parmesan cheese—Use sparingly as a seasoning.

Nonfat or low-fat frozen yogurt—an acceptable dessert

Almonds or hazelnuts (filberts)—for limited use in baking or sometimes as a garnish. These do contain fat, however, so use care.

Whole wheat flour—store in freezer.

Whole grain breads—preferably those without added fat and sugar. Store in the freezer if keeping past freshness date.

Skinned chicken breast fillets or turkey breast slices (4 or 5 ounces raw)—a ready convenience for quick cooking.

Ground turkey breast (skin-and fat-free)

More About Herbs

Trimming the fat is much easier when you rely on fresh and dried herbs. Both offer lots of flavor but no fat or cholesterol. The general rule of thumb when substituting fresh for dried herbs is to double the amount: dried herbs have a more intense flavor.

BASIL

Sweet, mild, clove-like flavor. Marries well with any dish that contains tomato: spaghetti, pizza, vegetable stew. Sprinkle on top of zucchini, eggplant, or yellow squash.

DILL

Fragrant and versatile best describe this feathery green. Toss with red potatoes or carrots. Mix with nonfat, plain yogurt to make a sauce for salmon or raw cucumber salad.

CILANTRO

Pungent, unusual flavor that gives spunk to Mexican salsa; a taste you'll either love or hate. Add it to soups and sauces in the last few minutes of cooking because it loses flavor when heated.

OREGANO

Strong, almost bitter herb that's ideal in Italian dishes. Try it in chili, or sprinkle over chicken.

TARRAGON

Distinctive, aromatic herb. Jazzes up chicken salad, soups, and meats like chicken or ham; common ingredient in flavored vinegars.

THYME

Known as the "stuffing herb"; add it to just about any meat dish, from lamb to chicken to beef. Adds a nice touch to cooked vegetables.

If you haven't used herbs and spices much in cooking, the following table might be helpful in deciding which ones to experiment with.

Aromatic Herbs and Spices

ALLSPICE
offers a cinnamon-nutmeg-clove flavor

ANISEED
tastes like licorice

CARDAMOM
tastes like a ginger-cinnamon mixture

CHERVIL
tastes like licorice

CINNAMON
has a musky, gentle flavor

CLOVES
taste woody, dark, and musky

DILL
adds a sweet flavor

FENNEL
tastes like licorice

FENUGREEK
has a bitter flavor

GARLIC
has a pungent, oniony taste

MACE
tastes like nutmeg

NUTMEG
has a woody, rich taste

PARSLEY
adds a woody flavor

ROSEMARY
has a hint of evergreen taste

SAGE
is earthy and musky

TARRAGON
tastes a little like licorice

THYME
is mild and fragrant

BASIL
is savory and sweet

BAY LEAF
is bittersweet

CORIANDER
tastes like lemon peel and sage

Sweet & Bittersweet Herbs & Spices

JUNIPER
is bittersweet and tastes
like pine

MARJORAM
is bittersweet and makes a
great salad herb

OREGANO
is bittersweet and has a
savory, lingering taste

PAPRIKA
can be mild or hot and
subtle or sweet

POPPY SEEDS
have a nutlike texture
and flavor

SAFFRON
is sweet, spicy, and mild

SESAME SEEDS
have a nutty flavor
and texture

VANILLA
has a sweet taste

Sharp, Peppery & Hot Herbs & Spices

CARAWAY
makes food taste richer

CAYENNE
tastes like ground red pepper

CHILI POWDER
is hot and adds a lot of
pizzazz

CUMIN
adds a yellowish color and
a pungent taste

CURRY
tastes pungent

GINGER
has a hot-sweet flavor

MINT
aromatic and clean taste

MUSTARD
adds a yellow color and a
hot, spicy taste

PEPPER
is hot when black or red,
milder when white

TURMERIC
tastes savory and spicy,
adds yellow color

Chapter 8

Dining Out With an Eye Toward Low Fat

Granted, it is harder to monitor fat content of meals when someone else is doing the cooking. But the growing array of lean listings at fast-food and family restaurants is making low-fat dining much simpler. Just look at all the new menu additions: broiled and grilled entrees, meatless main dishes, stir-fries, creamless sauces, fruit and vegetable salsas, frozen yogurt, and fresh-fruit sorbets.

Once you learn to decipher the menu lingo, it becomes easier to balance high-fat and low-fat choices so that you remain within recommended fat guidelines. For instance, if seafood or potatoes au gratin is a favorite dish, realize that these two words indicate a preparation technique that includes lots of butter and cheese. Balance that high-fat entree choice by choosing leaner side dishes. Maybe you can order a salad dressed with a splash of red wine vinegar rather than heavy dressing. For dessert try low-fat items like sherbet or fresh-fruit cocktail.

Nothing has to be totally off-limits, but it's best to select smaller portions of high-fat foods and indulge in them less frequently. Or consider sharing a particularly high-fat appetizer with several people. That way you can taste a dish without overindulging in fat. But above all become familiar with which foods are high in fat and which are low in fat. That way you can juggle selections accordingly.

Figuring Out Fast Food

Quick meals at a neighborhood fast-food restaurant need no longer be a high-fat, high-cholesterol, nutrition nightmare. Thanks to the arrival of leaner menu selections such as grilled chicken, broiled fish, and low-fat hamburgers, it's possible to grab a convenient meal without sabotaging attempts to limit fat. Here are a few pointers on how to keep fast-food dining low in fat.

▲ Opt for small, plain burgers instead of sandwiches with the works. Extras like cheese and special sauces are usually high in fat and calories.

▲ Leave the mayonnaise off large burgers and save about 150 calories. Skip the tartar sauce with fish; mayonnaise makes it high in fat. Better choices: catsup, mustard, seafood sauce, cocktail sauce.

▲ Skip the "extra crispy" fried chicken. Extra fat is what makes it crispier, and there can be as many as 100 calories more per piece. Peel off the skin to save even more fat.

▲ Satisfy a sweet tooth with low-fat frozen yogurt cones rather than a fried pie or hot fudge sundae.

▲ Enjoy pizza with vegetable toppings or lean ham instead of high-fat meats like sausage or pepperoni. Ask for half the cheese.

▲ Try salad as a side dish instead of french fries. Limit high-fat salad ingredients such as cheese, croutons, and sunflower seeds; choose a reduced-fat dressing.

▲ Select a baked potato and top it with vegetables from the salad bar or low-fat cottage cheese.

▲ Order cereals, English muffins with jam, bagels, and fruit juices for breakfast rather than sandwiches piled with eggs, sausage, and cheese.

▲ If you do go the big-burger-and-fries route on occasion, practice a little nutrition damage control. Eat grilled chicken or fish with pasta and a salad at the next meal.

Fat Content of Traditional Fast-Food Items

Item	Grams of Fat	Calories
Bacon cheeseburger	27	464
Burrito	14	448
Cheeseburger	14	295
Chili, 1 cup	8	254
English muffin (with butter)	6	189
Fish sandwich	23	431
French fries (20 to 25 in veg. oil)	12	235
French toast (5 sticks)	29	479
Fried chicken, 3 oz.	14	235
Hamburger	12	275
Hot dog	15	242
Nachos (6 to 8 with cheese)	19	345
Pancakes (3, with butter and syrup)	14	519
Pie (fruit, fried)	14	235
Pizza, cheese (1/8 of 12-inch)	3	140
Pizza, pepperoni (1/8 of 12-inch)	7	181
Potato chips (1 oz.)	10	148
Shake, vanilla, 10 oz.	8	314
Taco (6 oz. small)	11	183
Tuna salad sub sandwich (9 oz.)	28	584

Data from Pennington JAT. Bowes and Church's Food Values of Portions Commonly Used. 16th ed. Philadelphia: JB Lippincott Co; 1994.

Mastering Menu Terminology

For the most part terms used on menus tend to be descriptive of preparation techniques.

Terms That Signal High Fat Content

▲ creamed

▲ pan-fried

▲ buttery

▲ sauteed

▲ with gravy

▲ hollandaise sauce

▲ bernaise sauce

▲ au gratin

Terms That Signal Lighter Cooking

▲ grilled

▲ steamed

▲ poached

▲ broiled without butter

▲ braised

▲ blackened

If you're still in doubt about a certain item, don't hesitate to ask the server. Because nutrition is now on the curriculum at many culinary schools, many chefs are in tune to fat and cholesterol concerns. Some chefs employ registered dietitians to provide nutrition profiles for everything from appetizer to dessert.

Materials are provided by some American Heart Association (AHA) affiliates. The AHA works with restaurant owners in many cities to highlight lower-fat menu items. Call the local AHA office for free brochures or information about heart-healthy dining. Or look for special notes and symbols on menus that denote low-fat menu selections.

Sometimes making these ideas work in the real world is a major challenge. Picture yourself in a lovely restaurant, with your favorite dining companions, about to choose what you want for your evening meal.

The bread delivered before the meal is usually okay, but if you cover it with a pat or two of butter, you might be consuming a lot of calories before you've even ordered your dinner. One slice of French bread has about 80 calories and 1 gram of fat. One teaspoon of butter has 36 calories and 4 grams of fat. Put them together and you have a high-fat combination that doesn't carry many nutrients.

When you choose to have soup, order selections made with clear broths or tomato base instead of creamy styles. Be careful about soups like French onion, however. If it has a cheese topping, it carries about 100 calories per cup and about 8 grams of fat.

If you decide to have an appetizer, try a shrimp or a crab cocktail. Half a cup has about 65 calories with only about 1 gram of fat. A tablespoon of cocktail sauce adds only about 15 calories and no fat.

An even better choice of appetizer is a raw vegetable platter, as long as you are careful about adding the creamy dip that might come with it. While the most healthful choice is vegetables without dip, if you want the dip, put a small serving on your plate and limit your intake to that amount.

Here's a summary of basic tips to cover the rest of the meal:

▲ Watch out for anything described as creamed, breaded, or fried. Try to avoid anything dressed with mayonnaise; that means potato salad, coleslaw, or macaroni salad.

▲ Avoid ordering meat, poultry, or seafood portions larger than about 3 ounces cooked. (They usually come in portions of about 6 ounces, but before you start to eat, set half the portion aside. It will be just as good for tomorrow's lunch.)

▲ Order your meat, poultry, or seafood grilled, broiled without butter or added fat, or poached.

▲ If your entree is usually sauteed or simmered in cream or butter, ask that it be done in wine instead.

▲ Sauces and dressings can really be a challenge when you are trying to skim the fat, so order them on the side or ask that they be withheld. If you want to have some, use your teaspoon to portion out only the amount that your daily calorie and fat plan accommodates.

▲ On the side, load up on carbohydrates. Eat the rice, plain baked potato, vegetables, and beans.

▲ When they bring the dessert tray around, look for the fresh fruit and ask for the whipped cream on the side or ask for only a small dollop on top.

If you follow these simple suggestions, you should be able to limit your fat intake and still enjoy dining out.

Lighten Up at Lunch Time

Sandwiches mean lunch to many working people and students. Knowing how to fill those sandwiches to make them low-fat and healthful can mean the difference between a high-fat or low-fat lunch.

Suppose your choice is between a French-dip steak sandwich or a breast of turkey sandwich on wheat with spicy mustard and tomato slices. Which do you think is lower in fat? How about a chicken breast sandwich, hold the mayonnaise and butter, or a chicken-salad sandwich (which is about 48 percent of calories from fat)?

Better Sandwich Fillings

▲ Turkey or chicken breast slice

▲ Roast beef slices

▲ Tuna, chicken, shrimp, or crab salad, made with yogurt or reduced-calorie mayonnaise

▲ Low-fat or nonfat cheeses (less than 5 gm. fat per ounce)

Not-So-Good Choices

▲ Salami

▲ Polish sausage or liverwurst

▲ Bologna

▲ Chicken, tuna, or egg salad made with real mayonnaise

▲ Regular cheeses

If sandwiches are your preference, start with low-fat, high-in-fiber bread. Choose whole wheat or whole grain breads over croissants, crescent rolls, or white breads.

When you make your sandwich, add all the lettuce leaves, tomato slices, and onion slices you want. These add fewer than 10 calories each. Think about reducing or eliminating the mayonnaise. One tablespoon of mayonnaise adds 100 calories, 99 percent of which are from fat.

Mustard or catsup are better choices and often do a better job of adding flavor without fat. Yes, they do add a little sodium, but one teaspoon of mustard has only about 6 milligrams of sodium, while catsup has 170 milligrams. Don't overdo it; use a moderate amount.

When you order that lunch from the deli, think about passing on the potato salad, coleslaw, and potato chips. To accompany your sandwich, try fresh fruit, raw veggies, or a green salad (but watch the dressing!)

What about the salad bar? If this is a frequent lunch option for you, here are some guidelines to help you make wise choices.

Choose these salad options less often

2-tablespoon portions, unless otherwise noted

	Grams of fat	Calories
Lean ham, 1/3 cup, diced	5	70
Fried noodles, croutons	1	28
Coleslaw, 1/3 cup	7	120
Parmesan cheese	3	46
Chopped egg	1	16
Potato salad, 1/3 cup	3	128
Sunflower seeds	7	97
Macaroni salad, 1/3 cup	1	118
Cheddar cheese, grated	5	56
Bacon, crumbled, 1 tablespoon	2	27
Avocado, 1/4 whole	7	81
Black olives	2	25

Source: Pennington, J.A.T., Bowes & Church's Food Values of Portions Commonly Used, 16th Ed., Philadelphia, J.B. Lippincott, 1994.

Better salad ingredients

1/8-cup portions unless otherwise noted

	Grams of fat	Calories
Cauliflower, 1/3 cup	0	4
Carrot, grated	0	5
Strawberries, 1/3 cup	0	15-50
Pineapple, 1/3 cup	0	15-50
Melon pieces, 1/3 cup	0	20
Kidney beans	trace	27
Green peas	0	12
Tomato, 1/2 whole	0	12
Cucumber, 6 slices	0	2
Broccoli, 1/3 cup	0	8
Green pepper	0	4
Crab meat and shrimp, 1/3 cup	trace	40-60
Mushrooms	0	2
Garbanzo beans	0.5	21
Turkey, chicken breast, 1/3 cup	1	70-80

Source: Pennington, J.A.T., Bowes & Church's Food Values of Portions Commonly Used, 16th Ed., Philadelphia, J.B. Lippincott, 1994

Skim the Fat

Once you've made your salad choices, here's what you should know about salad dressings:

Use these salad dressings

Serving size = 2 Tablespoons

	Grams of fat	Calories
Nonfat yogurt, plain	0	16
Low-fat French dressing	1.8	44
Low-calorie Italian	1.5	16
Low-fat ranch	2	29
Low-fat yogurt, plain	0.5	18
Light sour cream	1	45

But try to pass on these full-fat choices

Mayonnaise-style dressings	10	114
Thousand Island	11	118
French	13	134
Russian	16	152
Italian	14	138
Bleu cheese	16	154
Ranch	12	114

Source: Pennington, J.A.T., Bowes & Church's Food Values of Portions Commonly Used, 16th Ed., Philadelphia, J.B. Lippincott, 1994

When choosing salad dressings, look for low-fat ones. Read labels and remember your goals. Even one tablespoon of dressing can make a great difference in the fat content of your salad. Making a lower-fat choice can mean a lot.

Plane Fare

Airline travelers can dine on low-fat meals simply by making their special request at least 24 hours before departure. Most major airlines are trimming the fat from regular menus, too. Fresh fruits and low-fat milk are turning up with regularity. Cereal or yogurt often replaces eggs and bacon for breakfast. Occasionally pretzels (1 gram of fat per ounce) stand in for peanuts (14 grams of fat per ounce) as a snack.

Ordering a special meal is relatively easy. Simply call the airline at least 24 hours ahead. If you're a frequent flyer, specify which meal you want and the airline will list it in your record for future flights.

Possibly the best choice on airlines is the fruit or seafood plate. These are served cold and are usually still flavorful, even if you are the last to be served on a flight. (This is usually the only inconvenience for travelers who have ordered a special meal. By the same token, special meals are sometimes delivered first, so be sure to identify yourself to the flight attendant to make delivery as easy as possible.)

The fruit plate can range from a simple array of fresh fruit to fruit with cottage cheese and yogurt with crackers. The seafood plate might be shrimp or seafood salad served with greens, dressing, and crackers. Most dressings are served on the side, which allows you better control over your fat intake.

The airlines are prepared to accommodate their health-conscious passengers these days, so don't hesitate to order your special meals ahead of time when you travel.

Skim the Fat

Chapter 9

Multicultural Dining

Tapping into the lean cuisine of other countries is easy once you become familiar with food ingredients and preparation techniques. Traditional Japanese restaurants win awards for the most low-fat selections: the emphasis is on vegetables, seafood, and rice. But all international cuisines have at least a few low-fat, high-flavor dishes to tempt the diner's taste buds. Master the basic task of learning low-fat ingredients and cooking techniques, and apply the principles to these popular international cuisines.

Chinese Dining

Lots of high-fat selections lurk among lower-fat fare. Watch out for stir-fries and sweet-and-sour dishes that contain deep-fat fried meats. Lemon chicken, for example, usually contains chicken that is first breaded and fried before being added to stir-fried vegetables.

Fried wontons, fried noodles, fried egg rolls, and egg foo yong are all on the high-fat list. The tip-off? The word "fried," of course. What's not so obvious, however, are choices like lobster sauce, which contains egg yolks; fried rice, which typically adds up to 400 calories a cup, 45 percent from fat; Peking duck; crispy fish (which is fried); any batter-dipped and fried shrimp or chicken, or fried dim sum. All of these are high in fat.

Chinese dining is a good way to practice fat balancing. If you order green pepper beef, where the meat comes in strips and measures about 3/4 cup, you have about 285 calories, 68 percent of them from fat. If you mix the dish with 1 1/2 cups of rice, the meal is now 28 percent calories from fat.

If you order something that is, say, about half chicken, tofu, or meat and the other half is vegetables, you need only add the same amount of rice as your stir-fry dish. Try broccoli with chicken over 1 1/4 cup rice and you have a low-fat meal. You can use this balancing technique with shrimp in black bean sauce, tofu with veggies, chicken in snow peas, or a choice of your own, just as long as some part of the main dish is vegetables.

Indian Dining

Almost a completely vegetarian cuisine, Indian meals favor vegetable combinations with lots of spice. Low-fat sauces made with yogurt often adorn chicken and vegetable entrees. Brown rice is predominantly featured. Watch out for dishes that feature coconut milk or cream. Remember that ghee is made from butter.

Indian food closely resembles Thai food, both in similarity of spices and ingredients. Curries are commonly served in both countries. They can be quite hot and spicy. Rice is a predominant feature of both cuisines. Basmati rice is a rice of choice in India, and it is frequently used in Indian restaurants in the

United States. This long-grained, aromatic rice is unique to India and is considered to be of premium quality.

Typical Indian cuisine uses ground spices, usually aromatic or fragrant spices like cardamom, coriander, cumin, cloves, and cinnamon. All of these are used in curry, a word which actually means "sauce" to the Indian people.

Frequently used cooking methods in Indian cuisine include stewing, frying, boiling, and steaming. Appetizers and breads are usually fried, and main dishes, stewed. Some traditional Indian cooking techniques predate ovens, so there is little food preparation done in an oven. The one exception is the tandoor, a clay oven that uses charcoal, which is still used today to prepare tandoori chicken and a few other baked dishes.

Among the healthful attributes of Indian food are its accent on carbohydrates and de-emphasis of protein. Basmati rice, almost all carbohydrate, is a main element. Breads are considered an important part of the meal, but you need to watch out for the fried varieties.

Legumes, including lentils and chick peas, are often found in entrees or side dishes, and are good sources of soluble fiber and protein. (Remember, soluble fiber is thought to lower blood cholesterol and triglycerides.)

Vegetables are incorporated into most Indian meals. They might be in curry dishes, biryani, and pullao (both these latter are based on basmati rice). The vegetables most commonly served are spinach, eggplant,

Low-fat Indian food choices include:

Lentil and chick-pea curries

Chicken and vegetables

Chicken rice pilaf

Basmati rice

Raita (cucumber and yogurt sauce)

Naan (bread baked in a tandoori oven)

Fruit and vegetable chutneys

cabbage, potatoes, and peas. Onions, green peppers, and tomatoes are often found in the stewed entrees.

Yogurt is frequently used in gravies and is usually the plain, low-fat variety, but it is good to ask to be sure. Protein choices are typically chicken or seafood, both low in fat. Rarely will any beef be found on a true Indian menu; the cow is considered sacred in India.

Indian cooking styles that are lower in fat are:

Tikka (pan roasted)

Cooked with or marinated in yogurt

Cooked with green vegetables

Cooked with onions, tomatoes, peppers, and/or mushrooms

Cooked with spinach

Baked

Masala

Tandoori

Cooked with curry (but be careful of the coconut milk)

Garnished with dried fruits

Higher fat Indian cooking styles are:

Fried

Dipped in batter

Dipped in chick-pea batter

Deep fried

Korma

Stuffed and fried

Creamy curry sauce (this one has coconut milk, for sure)

Ghee (made with butter)

Buttered, made with butter

Garnished with nuts

Italian Dining

Think pasta with red sauce instead of white (cream) sauce when dining Italian. Fried dishes like eggplant Parmesan are obvious fat sources. But large quantities of olive oil, cheese, and fatty meats like sausage and prosciutto turn low-fat pastas into high-fat meals.

In the pasta department, spaghetti is a good choice. If you want to cover your pasta, order the Marsala sauce, which is made with wine, or the marinara, made with tomatoes, onions, and garlic. It's the pesto and cream type sauces that are high in fat.

Other high-fat choices include manicotti or cannelloni rolls; two rolls have about 800 calories with 65 percent from fat and 300 to 600 milligrams of cholesterol. A better choice is stuffed ravioli or tortellini with Marinara sauce. A large serving of meat-filled ravioli with tomato sauce and a generous amount of cheese has about 700 calories, 42 percent from fat.

When we dine Italian in the United States, we often opt for pizza, something not always found on the menu in Italy. The less-fat choices are the vegetarian special or the cheese-only versions, which have about 28 to 32 percent of the calories from fat. Be careful how many slices you consume, however, since a pizza meal is difficult to balance when it comes to fat. You could order a dressing-free salad or bring a bag of carrot sticks from home.

Low-fat Italian food choices include:

Minestrone

Breadsticks

Pasta with red clam sauce

Pasta with marinara sauce

Chicken or veal cacciatore

Veal piccata

Italian ices

Cappuccino

Menu choices to shy away from when you visit the local Italian restaurant:

Alfredo

Carbonara

Saltimbocca

Parmigiana

Pancetta

Cooked in oil

Stuffed with cheese

Stuffed with ricotta

Prosciutto

Pecorino cheese (Romano)

In creamy sauce

Made with three
varieties of cheese

Egg and cheese batter

Fried

Veal sausage

Manicotti

Cannelloni

Ravioli

The better choices are:

Lightly sauteed with onions

Made with shallots

With peppers and
mushrooms

Artichoke hearts

Sun-dried tomatoes

Spicy marinara sauce

Tomato-based sauce,
marinara or cacciatore

Marsala sauce

Light red sauce

Light red-or-white wine
sauce

Light mushroom sauce

With capers

With herbs and spices

With garlic and oregano,
crushed tomatoes,
and spices

Florentine (spinach)

Grilled

Red or white clam sauce

Primavera (with vegetables,
but watch the sauce for
cream)

Lemon sauce

Piccata

Japanese Dining

Low-fat dishes that feature vegetables and condiment-size portions of chicken, seafood, and beef are staples at Japanese restaurants. Glazes and sauces are typically made with lean ingredients: broth, soy sauce (high in sodium), rice wine, sake.

But steer clear of tempura (battered and fried) foods. In addition to tempura, tonkatsu (deep fried pork), torikatsu (deep fried chicken), and katsudon (deep fried pork, onion, and egg) contain lots of fat and loads of sodium. Sodium increases even more if your entree is covered in sauce. One tablespoon of teriyaki sauce contains 690 milligrams of sodium, even though it has no fat and very few calories.

One word to look for on a Japanese menu is yakimono, which means broiled with little fat added. And rice is always a good choice for a low-fat, carbohydrate-rich filler.

Also, you might try sushi. Sushi is vinegared rice rolled up in several different ways, with seaweed or raw fish, or vegetables, or both. Even when an oily fish is used, it adds little fat to this interesting appetizer.

Tofu is often used in Japanese cooking. It can be incorporated in sauces and other foods without adding much fat. Four ounces of tofu, about 1/2 cup, total 94 calories, with about 6 grams of fat.

Low-fat Japanese food choices include:

Miso and bean soups

Most combinations of grilled meats or seafood (such as scallops with oriental vegetables)

Teriyaki chicken

Yosenabe

Sukiyaki

Udon (noodles)

Shabu shabu

Steamed rice

Rice noodles

Green tea

Mexican Dining

Basic ingredients in Mexican cuisine, such as corn, beans, tortillas, and tomatoes are low in fat. However, extras, including cheese, sour cream, and guacamole, can boost the fat content of Mexican meals to outrageous levels. Sidestep or limit these extras and watch out for fried tortilla shells and beans or other foods prepared with lard.

Low-fat Mexican food choices include:

Salsa

Gazpacho

Red beans and rice

Soft chicken tacos

Refried beans (no lard)

Taco salad (minus the fried shell)

Arroz con pollo (chicken and rice)

Fajitas

Burritos

Many Mexican restaurants are beginning to offer lower fat alternatives, such as low-fat sour cream. But you still need to be careful about guacamole. Its fat calories can add up very quickly.

If you choose to order a taco or tostada, try the chicken instead of beef and ask if you can have the tortilla steamed or baked instead of fried. Soft tortillas generally are a better choice than the crunchy ones.

If you want an enchilada, chicken again is probably your lowest-fat choice. Vegetables also are a healthful option, but once again, beware of frying.

Beans are an excellent source of fiber, and beans and rice provide an excellent and filling side dish. Bean burritos also are a healthful choice, while beef and bean combos tend to be much higher in fat.

If you enjoy a taco salad every now and again, skip the fried shell and pass on the sour cream and guacamole. Salsa makes an excellent dressing and saves significant amounts of fat.

French Dining

French food is not a particularly good choice for those of us who want to "skim the fat" from our diets. Almost every dish contains some eggs, butter, cream, or lots of salt, and many dishes include all of the above.

A cheese souffle, for example, is loaded with fat and cholesterol. A two-cup serving averages out at around 600 calories, with about 70 percent of calories from fat and almost 500 milligrams of cholesterol. Be very alert to the names of items and ask about the butter and cream content when you are in doubt.

Some better choices of French cuisine include anything without a sauce. Start off with a lean chicken breast or fish fillet. If it comes smothered in a sauce, ask for the sauce on the side. Hollandaise and Bernaise contain about 450 calories per half cup—almost all from fat. Bechamel sauce is made with milk, butter, and flour, and has more than 200 calories per half cup, most from fat.

French cooking is delicious, and French restaurants tend to be elegant. You certainly can enjoy them without sacrificing a healthful eating plan. Look for items like fish fillets poached in white wine or steamed seafood. Load up on vegetables and salad, with just a little dressing on the side.

Greek Dining

Meat, olive oil, butter, and creamy dressings are used in a lot of Greek cuisine. The meat is usually lamb, sometimes beef, slowly roasted on a spit. That's a good way to cook it, but portion sizes tend to be a problem with Greek restaurants. Splitting entrees may be an excellent way to enjoy Greek food without going overboard on calories and fat. Also, be careful of salad dressings, even the ones made from yogurt. They can still be high in fat.

The best Greek choices include:

Shish kabob made with lamb and vegetables and roasted on a spit

Plaki (fish cooked with tomatoes, onions, and garlic)

Pilaf (rice)

Bread (hold the butter)

On the appetizer list, try to avoid babaganoosh (an eggplant appetizer made with fat), Kibbeh (lamb and butter), and tyropita and spanokopita (pies that are full of fat).

The Greek taste treat that rates in the "very high fat" category is baklava, probably the richest dessert ever created. It's made with butter, nuts, which are high in fat, honey, and sugar.

What are the good choices? Shish kabob made with lamb and vegetables and roasted on a spit; Plaki, fish cooked with tomatoes, onions, and garlic; and rice pilaf and bread, but hold the butter.

Thai Dining

Thai food, generally speaking, fits well into a healthy eating program when we want to "skim the fat." It is light on fats, meats, and sauces, and heavy on vegetables, noodles, and rice. It may be, overall, a healthier choice than Chinese food, to which it is quite similar.

Thai food, as a matter of fact, is often compared to Chinese food because of the stir-fry cooking technique it employs, the predominant role of rice, and the use of similar ingredients: shrimp, chicken, onions, and mushrooms, to name a few. But Thai food tastes substantially different from Chinese because of the spices used. In Thai food, the quality is hot and spicy, achieved through the use of coriander, cumin, cardamom, cinnamon, and several more spices, all blended into what Americans know as curry, which is also typical of Indian fare.

The manner of cooking, where the foods are cut up into small pieces and quickly cooked by stir-frying in a wok, again is sim-

Avoid items with the following labels—all high in fat.

Sizzling

Deep fried

Fried

Crispy

Until golden brown

Stir-fried

Topped with peanuts, peanut sauce

Peanuts, cashews

Curry sauce (often made with coconut milk)

Made with coconut milk

Eggplant (usually fried)

Golden brown duck

Instead, choose items that are:

Sauteed

Broiled, boiled, or steamed

Braised

Barbecued

Charbroiled

Made in basil sauce, basil, or with sweet basil leaves

Made in lime sauce

Made in chili sauce or with crushed dried chili

Served in a hollowed-out pineapple

Made with fish sauce

Made with napa, bamboo shoots, black mushrooms,
ginger, and garlic on a bed of mixed vegetables

ilar to the Chinese style. But the high-sodium soy sauce is replaced with nam pla, or fish sauce made from dried fish and spices. Even though there is some fat in the cooking technique, the foods are not immersed in it. And with the quick, wok-cooking style, less fat is absorbed into the food.

On the less positive side, coconut milk is often used in Thai cuisine, and unfortunately, it is loaded with fat. Beware of menu choices bearing coconut milk, like the curry-sauced entrees.

Rice is the usual accompaniment to the Thai meal, and that lends itself well to fat balancing. Therefore, the rule for Chinese cuisine can be aptly applied here. And Thai chefs do not add salt to the rice when they cook it. The other starch common in Thailand is called pad thai, a noodle dish.

The traditional Thai main meal consists of soup, rice, a curry dish, vegetables, a salad, and several sauces. The most common protein foods on menus in Thai restaurants are seafood—shrimp, scallops, squid, and clams. There are also lots of chicken and duck offerings. Be careful about choosing duck, which is naturally high in fat.

You can also feel good about eating most vegetable entrees. Try the vegetable boat (string beans, asparagus, zucchini, onions, and mushrooms stir-fried in Thai spices), or the Pad jay (a combination of napa, celery, onions, carrots, mushrooms, and bean sprouts, topped with a sauce of Thai spices). The rice and noodle dishes can help you balance the fat, but watch out for the fried rice varieties. Ask for the rice steamed.

Chapter 10

Becoming a Supermarket Fat Sleuth

Eating for heart health begins in the supermarket. To make the right choices here it is important to read labels to determine the fat content of your favorite foods.

The definitions below will help clear up confusion about the ingredient terminology on food labels. And the two charts that follow will give you some guidance on how to choose margarines and oils.

A Supermarket Glossary

Hydrogenated fat—Commercially processed fat or oil that is exposed to hydrogen to make it become more solid. Hydrogenation increases the amount of saturated fatty acids found in a fat. Margarines and vegetables shortenings vary greatly in the degree of hydrogenation. A soft tub margarine will have less saturated fat than a stick margarine.

Partially hydrogenated fat—Commercially processed liquid oil that doesn't undergo complete hydrogenation. It is less solid than completely hydrogenated fat. During hydrogenation some polyunsaturated fats are converted to monounsaturated, and some monounsaturated fats are converted to saturated.

Monoglyceride or diglyceride—Two kinds of fat used in tiny quantities by food manufacturers because of their ability to act as emulsifying agents and prevent foods from separating.

Fat Profiles of Vegetable Oils			
Oil type	Polyunsaturated fatty acids	Monounsaturated fatty acids	Saturated fatty acids
Safflower	75%	12%	9%
Sunflower	66%	20%	10%
Corn	59%	24%	13%
Soybean	58%	23%	14%
Cottonseed	52%	18%	26%
Canola	33%	55%	7%
Olive	8%	74%	13%
Peanut	32%	46%	17%
Palm	9%	37%	49%
Coconut	2%	6%	86%
Palm kernel	2%	11%	81%

Adapted from National Heart, Lung, and Blood Institute. Facts About Cholesterol. Bethesda, Md: US Dept of Health and Human Services, Public Health Service, National Institutes of Health, 1987.

Because food companies use such minute amounts of these oils, they are not a large source of saturated fat in most diets.

Tropical oil—Vegetable oils that contain large quantities of saturated fat. The three oils that make up this list are coconut, palm, and palm kernel. Manufacturers still use tiny quantities of these oils in some bakery products and candies because tropical oils help to extend product shelf life and do not turn rancid.

Choosing a Vegetable Oil

Even if you understand the concept of saturated and unsaturated fat, choosing a vegetable oil might seem tricky. A product like canola oil advertises that it is the lowest in saturated fat of all vegetable oils. Olive oils are touted for their high monounsaturated fat content. And oils like corn, sunflower, and safflower boast of a high concentration of polyunsaturated fat. Which product is best?

Don't worry over the small differences in types of fat. It really isn't important whether the unsaturated fat is mainly monounsaturated or polyunsaturated. The important point is to remember that oil is fat and to aim for moderation.

Substitutes for Fat

No discussion of low-fat eating is complete without some mention of a new category of low-fat supermarket foods—foods made with fat substitutes. These substances are being used with increasing regularity. Most of the substitutes currently on the market carry fewer calories than their full-fat counterparts but are not calorie free.

Fat replacements must be approved by the Food and Drug Administration (FDA) before they can be added to any food. The following paragraphs briefly explain what kind of substitutes manufacturers are using or plan to use in the future. Keep in mind that foods made with fat substitutes can still be high in calories.

Carbohydrate- or starch-based substitutes—Food companies have been using gums and modified food starches (made from potatoes, tapioca, or cornstarch) for years as thickeners in foods like ice creams and salad dressing. Now that fat-free foods are all the rage, manufacturers are using old technology to reformulate new reduced-fat products. Scientists have also developed a fat substitute made from oat flour that is currently being used to make extra-lean ground beef.

Protein-based fat substitutes—Several food companies are working to formulate fat replacements from egg white and milk proteins. One of the first fat substitutes to gain approval by the FDA was made using these two protein foods. The protein-based substitute cannot be used for frying, but it is already helping to lower the fat content of frozen confections and refrigerated food products.

Fat-based substitutes—It seems odd that a fat substitute could be made from fat. Yet, scientists are chemically altering fatty acids in the lab to come up with substances that taste like fat yet are not digested or absorbed by the body.

Choosing a Margarine Product

With the plethora of margarines, spreads, and butter-margarine blends on the market, it can take hours to examine nutrition labels and decide the right product for you. If you don't have time for precise comparison, a few general rules of thumb can help.

Softer, tub margarines have less saturated fat than the stick varieties. Spreads are margarines to which water has been added. They contain less fat, but the proportion of saturated to unsaturated fat is not that different from regular margarines.

Butter-margarine blends contain less saturated fat than butter but more saturated fat than margarine. All of these products, even an occasional pat of butter, can work into a low-fat diet. Just remember to use fats sparingly.

As we mentioned earlier, margarines are often hardened by a process called hydrogenation, which makes them more versatile. During the hydrogenation process, some of the fats are changed to a material called trans fatty acids. Although there has been some discussion about whether trans fatty acids play a role in health, there is little evidence to suggest that current levels of consumption of trans fatty acids need to be changed.

Nutrient Comparison of Butters, Margarines, and Spreads

Serving size: 1 tablespoon

Product	Calories	Total fat (gm.)	Polyun- saturated- fat (gm.)	Saturated fat	Cholesterol (mg.)
Butter					
Stick	108	12	0.5	7.6	33
Whipped	81	9	0.3	5.7	24
Margarine					
Liquid, corn oil	100	11	6.0	2.0	0
Tub, corn oil	102	11	4.5	2.1	0
Tub, safflower	102	11	6.3	1.2	0
Stick, corn oil	102	11	2.4	1.8	0
Stick, soybean	102	11	3.0	2.4	0
Diet, corn oil	51	6	2.4	0.9	0
Butter-margarine blend					
(40% butter)	90	11	2.0	5.0	5
Spread with					
sweet cream	76	8	3.5	3.2	1

Source: Pennington, J.A.T., Bowes & Church's Food Values of Portions
Commonly Used, 16th Ed., Philadelphia, J.B. Lippincott, 1994.

The Importance of Reading Labels

Do you think that a food labeled "low-fat" or "nonfat" is one you can eat in unlimited quantities? Do you understand the definition of "light" or "lite"? Once packaged foods were required only to have their name on the package. But times have changed and the growing trend toward health consciousness has led to a nutrition label that affords the consumer more and better information.

The most recent changes to the food label are the result of the Nutrition Labeling and Education Act, passed in 1990 and implemented by the FDA in May of 1994. The law creates an entirely new food labeling system that appears on virtually all packaged foods. (Exempt foods include food sold by a small business or on site; vending machine foods; coffee, tea, and spices; small packaged items; fresh fruits and vegetables; and raw meat, poultry, and fish.) Many supermarkets are voluntarily posting or making available nutrient information for meat, poultry, fish, and produce. Look for posters, shelf tags, or brochures containing the Nutrition Facts information.

The new standards in food labeling provide consumers with more complete, informative, and easy-to-understand facts about individual foods than ever before. "Nutrition Facts" include information on serving sizes, calories, calories from fat, total fat, saturated fat, cholesterol, sodium, complex carbohydrates, dietary fiber, sugars, protein, vitamin A and C, calcium, and iron. Daily values for the nutrients show how the subject food fits into an overall daily diet.

Daily values are based on reference 2000 calorie and 2500 calorie diets. These are used to represent an average for healthy people: 2000 calories for healthy women, young children, or older adults; 2500 calories for men, pregnant women, and teenagers. Now you may not think you eat and drink 2000 calories in a day, but that's the actual average for American women.

Sample Food Label

Nutrition Facts

Serving Size 1/2 cup (114 g)
Servings Per Container 4

Amount Per Serving

Calories 260   Calories from Fat 120

	% Daily Value*
Total Fat 13 g	**20%**
Saturated Fat 5 g	**25%**
Cholesterol 30 mg	**10%**
Sodium 660 mg	**28%**
Total Carbohydrate 31 g	**11%**
Dietary Fiber 0 g	**0%**
Sugars 5 g	
Protein 5 g	

Vitamin A 4% • Vitamin C 2%
Calcium 15% • Iron 4%

*Percent Daily Values are based on a 2,000 calorie diet. Your daily values may be higher or lower depending on your calorie needs:

		Calories	2,000	2,500
Total Fat	Less than		65 g	80 g
Sat Fat	Less than		20 g	25 g
Cholesterol	Less than		300 mg	300 mg
Sodium	Less than		2400 mg	2400 mg
Total Carbohydrate			300 g	375 g
Dietary Fiber			25 g	30 g

Calories per gram:

Fat 9 • Carbohydrate 4 • Protein 4

The standard serving size and the number of servings in a package are listed here.

Total calories and those calories from fat are listed here.

% Daily Values indicate how a serving of this food fits into the overall diet. Values are based on a 2,000 calorie diet.

On some packages, Daily Values are listed for both a 2,000 calorie and a 2,500 calorie diet. Your own nutrient needs may be more or less than the Daily Values on the label. A registered dietitian (RD) can show you how to calculate your personal Daily Values.

This information reminds us how many calories are in one gram of a fat, a carbohydrate, or a protein.

Let's say, for example, that you're figuring your fat intake. If your breakfast foods make up 40 percent of the recommended daily fat intake, and your lunch adds another 30 percent, you probably won't want to choose foods for dinner that exceed 30 percent. Reading the Percent Daily Values on the labels helps you choose foods that add up to, but don't go over, the recommended total daily intake.

At the bottom of the label, the total recommended daily values appear (not just the percentages) for other nutrients so you can get an idea of the total amounts required. Use these figures as your guide when you select foods to fit into your personal daily food plans.

Standardized Serving Sizes

Check the Nutrition Facts panel on some of your favorite foods and you may be surprised at how few (or how many!) grams of fat a serving contains. That's because the serving size is now based on the amount people usually eat of that product. What causes the surprise is that the new standard serving size is not necessarily the amount you plan to eat. The lesson here is to always compare the label serving size with the amount you actually eat. One thing that is easier is comparing similar products without doing a lot of mental arithmetic. No more can one brand of macaroni and cheese say one serving is equivalent to 3/4 cup while another brand says one serving is 1/2 cup. All similar foods must follow the same serving size requirements.

Ingredient Listing

Another important thing you can do is read a product's list of ingredients. Reading the fine print tells the truth about the contents of the package. Ingredients are listed in order, and the ingredient present in the largest amount by weight is listed first. Other ingredients are listed in descending order according to weight.

Additives must also be listed, and if artificial colors are used, the manufacturer must list FDA-certified color additives by name. Colors exempt from certification, like caramel, paprika, and beet juice, can simply be called "artificial colors."

Products with "standards of identity," that meant their recipes were defined by law, used to be able to omit an ingredient list. Today even they are subject to the new food labeling law. You will now find an ingredient list on such things as catsup, macaroni, jelly, and orange juice.

Health Claims

The FDA now allows manufacturers to make certain claims linking the effects of a food or nutrient to a disease or health-related condition. Only claims supported by scientific evidence are allowed. Claims can be used only under certain conditions, such as when the food is an adequate source of the appropriate nutrients.

The claims may show a relationship between:

▲ a diet with enough calcium and a lower risk of osteoporosis

▲ a diet low in total fat and a reduced risk of some cancers

▲ a diet low in saturated fat and cholesterol and a reduced risk of coronary heart disease

▲ a diet rich in fiber-containing grain products, fruits, and vegetables and a reduced risk of some cancers

▲ a diet rich in fruits, vegetables, and grain products that contain fiber and a reduced risk of coronary heart disease

▲ a diet low in sodium and a reduced risk of high blood pressure

▲ a diet rich in fruits and vegetables and a reduced risk of some cancers.

▲ a diet with enough folic acid and a reduced risk of neural tube defects in offspring.

Consumers can use these claims to identify foods with desirable nutritional qualities. A reference to the claim may appear on the front label, but the claim itself may appear elsewhere on the label.

What Do All Those Terms Mean?

Certain terms have become so common that it's hard to tell what they really mean. New strict labeling laws and definitions have been set by the FDA and have to be followed by manufacturers. Here's a rundown of what various terms mean (in these definitions, "per serving" refers to reference amounts set by the government):

Reduced, less, fewer—These apply to foods that have been altered to contain at least 25 percent less of whatever it is that's reduced. For example, a package might say "reduced fat," "less sodium," or "fewer calories." The claim must include the percent of difference and the name of the product it's being compared with. If the regular product already meets "low" standards, the new product can't make "reduced" claims.

Lite, light—These apply to foods that contain at least one-third less calories or 50 percent less fat than the regular product. It can also mean foods that have half the sodium content of the reference product. Other references to lite or light can refer to color, breading, or texture, but this should be noted on the label.

High, rich in, excellent source—These terms refer to foods containing 20 percent or more of the Daily Value for that nutrient in a serving. For example, "high in fiber," "rich in protein," or "excellent source of calcium."

Good source, contains, provides—These can be stated on a label if a food contains from 11 to 19 percent more of the Daily Value for the specific nutrient in a serving. For example, "good source of iron," "contains fiber," or "provides vitamin C."

More—This refers to any food that has 10 percent more than the Daily Value per serving of a specific nutrient compared with the regular product. Dissimilar products can also be compared, such as frozen yogurt and ice cream.

Free—Products that say this have insignificant amounts of calories, fat, saturated fat, cholesterol, sodium, and/or sugar. Other synonyms for the term "free" are "no," "zero," "negligible source of," "dietarily insignificant source of," or "without." Examples are:

▲ Calorie free—must contain less than 5 calories per serving

▲ Cholesterol free—must have less than 2 milligrams of cholesterol and 2 grams or less of saturated fat per serving.

▲ Fat free—contains less than 0.5 grams of fat per serving

▲ Sugar free—must have less than 0.5 grams of sugar per serving.

Low, little, few—These refer to products that don't exceed dietary guidelines for calories, fat, saturated fat, cholesterol, and/or sodium. Examples are:

▲ Low fat—contains 3 grams or less per serving

▲ Low saturated fat—has 1 gram or less per serving, with no more than 15 percent of calories per serving coming from saturated fat

▲ Low sodium—contains 140 milligrams or less per serving

▲ Very low sodium — has 35 milligrams or less per serving

▲ Low cholesterol—contains 20 milligrams or less per serving

▲ Low calorie—has 40 calories or less per serving

Lean, extra lean—These apply to the fat content of meats, poultry, and seafood or fish. Examples are:

▲ Lean—contains less than 10 grams of fat, 4.5 grams or less of saturated fat, and less than 95 milligrams of cholesterol per serving.

▲ Extra lean—has less than 5 grams of fat, less than 2 grams of saturated fat, and less than 95 milligrams of cholesterol per serving (per 100 grams of the product's weight).

Enriched, fortified—These apply to foods that have been nutritionally altered to increase the Daily Value of one or more nutrients by at least 10 percent.

Percent fat free—Foods with this claim must meet the standards for low fat because people assume they can be included in a low-fat diet. The claim must also reflect the amount of fat present in 100 grams of the food. For example, if a food contains 3 grams of fat per 75 grams of weight, it's "96-percent fat free." Because these claims are based on weight and not on calories from fat, they can be very confusing. Be sure to check the label for calories from fat and the total grams of fat.

Healthy—Individual foods with this claim must meet the standards for low-fat and low-saturated fat. In addition, the individual food must not exceed 60 milligrams of cholesterol and 360 milligrams of sodium per serving. And at least 10 percent of the Daily Value for vitamin A, vitamin C, iron, calcium, fiber, or protein must be provided in one serving. For main dish and meal products, more cholesterol (up to 90 milligrams) and sodium (up to 600 milligrams) per serving are allowed, but the other standards remain the same.

Chapter 11

Basic Low-Fat Cooking Techniques

Saving Flavor

Professional chefs say that cooking with less fat doesn't necessarily spell disaster as far as taste is concerned. Over the years they've picked up a few tricks of the trade. But these are nothing that the home cook can't master. All you need is to have the right ingredients on hand. Then start by employing flavor enhancers: herbs, spices, and flavorful liquids.

In professional cooking, liquids such as lemon and orange juices, flavored vinegars (red wine, balsamic, raspberry, apple cider), and wines are used liberally in everything from sauces to soups to main dishes. Chefs depend on these items to add the finishing touch to prepared foods. You'll notice that the common thread between the liquids is that they are all acidic in nature.

It might seem that adding something acidic could overpower a dish. Ironically, it does just the opposite. Used in small amounts, wines, citrus juices—lemon, lime, and orange—and vinegars tend to round out flavor, offering a balance between salty, sweet, and bitter tastes. A splash of lemon juice, for instance, helps bring out the flavor of steamed vegetables like broccoli or asparagus.

Citrus juices in general help soften the strong taste of grilled foods, particularly chicken and fish. Adding fresh or dried herbs and spices rounds out the flavor even more.

Tricks of the Trade

Skimming the fat in your recipes means more than just using leaner ingredients. It also means using healthful cooking techniques and tools. Here are some quick tips:

1. Use low- and no-fat cooking methods, like steaming, poaching, stir-frying, broiling, grilling, microwaving, baking, and roasting as alternatives to frying.

2. Get a good quality set of no-stick saucepans, skillets, and baking pans so you can saute and bake without adding fat.

3. Try no-stick vegetable sprays or 1 to 2 tablespoons of defatted broth, water, juice, or wine to replace cooking oil.

4. Be aware that fat-free or reduced-fat cheeses have slightly different cooking characteristics than their fattier counterparts, so they don't melt as smoothly. To overcome this, shred these cheeses very finely. When making sauces and soups, toss the cheese with a small amount of flour, cornstarch, or arrowroot.

5. Trim all visible fat from steaks, chops, roasts, and other meat cuts before preparing them.

6. Replace one-quarter to one-half the ground meat or poultry in a casserole or meat sauce with cooked brown rice, bulgur, couscous, or cooked and chopped dried beans tol skim the fat and add fiber.

7. Deciding to remove the skin from poultry before or after cooking depends upon your cooking method. Skin helps prevent roasted or baked cuts from drying out, and studies have shown that the fat from the skin doesn't penetrate the meat during cooking. However, if you do leave the skin on, make sure any seasonings you've applied go under the skin or you'll lose the flavor when the skin is removed.

8. Skim and discard the fat from hot soups and stews, or chill the soup or stew and skim off the solid fat that forms on top.

9. Use pureed cooked vegetables, like carrots, potatoes, or cauliflower, to thicken soups and sauces instead of cream, egg yolks, or a butter and flour roux. Also, try using soft tofu to thicken sauces.

10. Select "healthier" fats when you need to add fat to a recipe. That means replacing butter, lard, or other highly saturated fats with oils such as canola, olive, safflower, sunflower, corn, and others that are low in saturates. Remember, it takes just a few drops of a very flavorful oil, such as extra-virgin olive oil, dark sesame, walnut, or garlic oil, to really perk up a dish, so go easy.

11. Skim the fat where you won't miss it, but keep the characteristic flavor of fatty ingredients like nuts, coconut, chocolate chips, and bacon by reducing the quantity you use by 50 percent. For example, if a recipe calls for 1 cup of walnuts, use 1/2 cup instead.

12. Toast nuts and spices to enhance their flavor, then chop them finely so they can be more fully distributed through the food.

13. If sugar is the primary sweetener in a fruit sauce, beverage, or other dish that is not baked, scale the amount down by 25 percent. Instead of using 1 cup of sugar, use 3/4 cup. If you add a pinch of cinnamon, nutmeg, or allspice, you'll increase the perception of sweetness without adding calories.

One word of caution: Be careful when cutting back on the amount of sugar in cakes, cookies, or other baked goods. Many times reducing sugar will affect the texture or the volume.

14. In baked goods, add pureed fruit instead of fat. One of the reasons fat is included in baked products is to make them moist. The high concentration of natural sweetness in pureed fruit will actually help hold on to the water moisture during the baking process.

Fat has flavor, but so does fruit. Fat adds liquid volume and moisture to bread or cake batter, but so does fruit. So when making this substitution, if the recipe calls for 1/2 cup of fat, simply add 1/2 cup of pureed fruit. Try applesauce in apple bran muffins or cakes. Pureed crushed pineapple works well in pineapple upside down cake.

Dark-colored fruits, like blueberries and prunes, are best used in dark-colored batters. Lighter colored fruits, like pears or applesauce, can be added to almost any batter without changing its color. Adding yellow-orange fruits, such as pureed peaches or apricots, can often add an appetizing yellowish crumb.

Pears and apples can be used nearly universally in baking because their taste is very mild and unnoticeable. Apricots, prunes, and pineapple add a much stronger flavor. Bananas and peaches are somewhere in the middle, adding a little flavor, but never overwhelming. And here's a secret: if you don't have a food processor to use to puree your own fruit, try using baby food. It is already pureed, has very mild flavor, and usually is made without sugar.

15. Beat egg whites until soft peaks form before incorporating them into baked goods. This will increase the volume and tenderness.

16. Make a simple fat-free "frosting" for cakes or bar cookies by sprinkling the tops lightly with powdered sugar.

17. Increase the fiber content and nutritional value of dishes by using whole-wheat flour for at least half of the all-purpose white flour. For cakes and other baked products that require a light texture, use whole-wheat pastry flour, available in some well-stocked supermarkets.

18. Vegetables can be fat replacements in other recipes, too. Try:

▲ Adding baby carrot puree, roasted red pepper puree, or mashed potatoes to your pasta sauce to replace olive oil.

▲ Replacing some of the fat in nut breads or cakes like carrot cake or zucchini bread with vegetable purees or juices like carrot juice or pumpkin puree.

▲ Substituting pureed green peas for half the amount of mashed avocado in guacamole or other dips.

▲ Replacing fat in soups, sauces, muffins, or cakes with mashed yams or sweet potatoes.

▲ Using white potatoes to thicken lower-fat milks in cream soups and bisques.

▲ Substituting a layer of vegetables in your favorite lasagna to replace meat or sausage.

▲ Topping your pizza with vegetables instead of meat.

Cooking Techniques for Cooking Leaner

Use cooking techniques that do not require fat whenever you can. When you are sauteing, however, you might want to try experimenting with fat replacements.

For cooking, try:

Low-sodium chicken, beef, or vegetable broth

Fruit juices

Flavored vinegars

Nonfat or light sour cream (to add creaminess to a gravy or sauce)

Plain water

Wine or beer

For baking, try:

Nonfat or light cream cheese

Nonfat or light sour cream

Flavored low-fat or nonfat yogurts

Fruit juice or fruit purees

Liquor or liqueurs (sherry, whiskey, orange, and coffee flavored liqueurs)

Evaporated skim milk

Don't be afraid to add less fat than the recipe calls for. In many cases, you can cut the amount of added butter or margarine in half and not miss it at all. You don't have to add any of the fat called for in cake and brownie mixes. Just remember to add a nonfat liquid in its place. Make a note of how much fat you can leave out of a recipe on your recipe card or in your books. Experiment by cutting the butter, margarine, or oil in half, then reduce it a little more each time you make the recipe.

Some Cooking Techniques and Terms

Al Dente: In Italian, *al dente* means "to the tooth"; in cooking it has a similar meaning—"crisp to the teeth", "resistant to the bite", or "cooked but still firm." Properly cooked pasta is a perfect example of al dente. The technique is also critical to well-made Chinese and Japanese dishes.

In addition to those foods that are best enjoyed before that bit of firmness is lost, grains and vegetables that are to be reheated or finished with a second stage of cooking should be slightly underdone initially, since they will continue to cook.

Cooking times vary according to the size and thickness of an item. For example, angel hair pasta will cook faster than fettuccine, julienned vegetables will cook faster than those left in larger pieces. Ripeness and quality also affect cooking times.

Vegetables that are to be cooked together should be cut in similar shapes and thicknesses. Those of varying sizes should be cooked separately, for they will cook at different rates.

Baking: This should always be done in a preheated oven because the heat will seal and prevent juices from escaping from foods and thus keep foods from drying out. For low-fat baking, a nonstick pan is best, but you can also use a pan lightly sprayed with vegetable oil. If your pan is sprayed too heavily, the extra fat should be wiped off. Waxed paper can be used to line molds or baking sheets that are not nonstick; the paper should be peeled off right after baking.

Braising: Braising and stewing are very similar, except that braising uses less liquid. When braising meat, the meat is slowly browned to develop color and flavor and then slowly cooked over low heat with a small amount of liquid in a pan with a tight cover.

For braising vegetables, cut them into uniform pieces to ensure even cooking. Partially cover the vegetables with liquid. Cover the pot and place it over a low to medium heat to prevent burning.

Using vegetable stock or wine adds to the flavor of vegetables. If you are braising a wide variety of vegetables, such as onions, carrots, celery, and leeks, you may not need to start with a stock because the vegetables will provide enough flavor of their own.

If you are cooking with water, add dried herbs at the same time you add the vegetables. Fresh herbs should be added toward the end of cooking; they have a tendency to lose flavor with prolonged cooking. Salt should also be added toward the end of cooking because saltiness becomes concentrated as the liquid evaporates during cooking. If you plan to use the braising liquid as a sauce and you find the flavor weak, strain the liquid away from the vegetables once they have been cooked. Then return it to a high heat and boil it to reduce the liquid and concentrate the flavor. Once the sauce is reduced, add fresh herbs, salt, pepper, and any thickening agents.

Grilling: This technique retains all the juices and flavor of food because it seals them in with dry heat. Use a nonstick grill and make sure it is clean and very hot before placing the meat or vegetables on it. Temperature and time depend on the type of meat or vegetable used. Different vegetables grilled together should be cut to the same thickness to ensure equal cooking time. Salt should be used only at the end of cooking, if at all. Remember, salt draws the moisture out of the food.

Parboiling or blanching: Parboiling or blanching is a way of partially cooking ingredients. Blanching is also done to extract bitterness from strongly flavored vegetables. Dry beans can be blanched as an alternative to soaking them overnight, which has the added advantage of extracting some of the elements in beans that cause flatulence.

To blanch beans, use ten times the amount of water to the amount of beans. Rinse and pick over the beans, then place them in cold water. Bring them to a boil, boil for 6 minutes, and finally, rinse and refresh under cold water before continuing with the recipe.

Blanching should always be done in a large amount of lightly salted boiling water. The salt can be omitted, but it does help to retain the colors of vegetables.

Green vegetables, in particular, contain elements that when subjected to heat change color and texture. Therefore, when blanching green vegetables, take the following steps:

1. Use a nonreactive pot—enameled or stainless steel. Bring the water to a rolling boil. Do not cover. Taste often to determine doneness.

2. Once cooked, the vegetables should be drained and submerged in a large amount of ice cold water to stop the cooking process.

Blanching times for some vegetables

Vegetable	Duration
Carrot, julienned	2 minutes
Celery stalk, julienned	2 minutes
Fennel bulb, julienned	2 minutes
Green beans (2-inch lengths)	1 minute
Green onions	30 seconds
Green peas, fresh	1 minute
Leek, julienned	30 seconds
Mushrooms, julienned	30 seconds
Snow peas	1 minute
Spinach	10 seconds
Summer squash	1 minute

Roasting: This is another way of cooking with dry heat. It is used for large cuts of meat, such as roasts, or whole birds. Roasting requires more time but very little attention. If a roasting rack is used, fat drains off during cooking.

Steaming: Like blanching, steaming, used mainly to cook vegetables, seals foods with a moist heat and helps to retain their nutrients, flavor, and texture. The water should be at a full boil to produce a high heat and full steam, but kept below the steaming rack and not in contact with the food. Watch the level of water carefully and add more water as needed.

Recipe Make-Overs

Once you commit to a low-fat lifestyle, don't feel compelled to throw away favorite recipes. With a little bit of remodeling, baked goods, meat pies, and cheesy casseroles can be made lower in fat. To start, run down the ingredient list and mark all the fatty ingredients: butter, oil, cheese, cream, meats.

With the exception of baked goods, it is feasible to cut butter and oils by one third to one half in most recipes. It is often better to replace rather than cut back on fat in baked goods because fat affects their texture. (See pages 129-130 for more information on replacing fat in baked goods.)

Next, replace fatty meats and full-fat cheeses with lean or lower-fat varieties. To give you an idea of how to reshape a recipe, here's a revamped traditional turkey pot pie. Notice the before-and-after nutrient profiles. With just a few simple changes, fat content is cut nearly in half without dramatically changing the taste. Net savings per serving: 17 grams of total fat, 16 grams of saturated fat, and 75 milligrams of cholesterol.

Turkey Pot Pies

BEFORE:
TRADITIONAL RECIPE PER SERVING
CALORIES 590, TOTAL FAT 38.8 GRAMS,
SATURATED FAT 19.3 GRAMS,
CHOLESTEROL 110 MILLIGRAMS

AFTER:
MODIFIED RECIPE PER SERVING
CALORIES 440, TOTAL FAT 21.9 GRAMS
SATURATED FAT 3.5 GRAMS,
CHOLESTEROL 35 MILLIGRAMS

Lower Fat Turkey Pot Pies

4 servings, 1 pot pie each

Pastry

1 cup flour
1/4 teaspoon salt
2 tablespoons water
1/4 cup oil (replaces 1/3 cup lard in traditional recipe)

Filling

1/3 cup diced potatoes
1/3 cup sliced carrots
1/3 cup frozen green peas
1/4 cup chopped celery
1 tablespoon chopped onion
1/2 cup boiling water
2 tablespoons soft margarine
(replaces 1/4 cup butter)
1/4 cup flour
1/2 teaspoon salt
1/8 teaspoon pepper
1/8 teaspoon poultry seasoning
1 1/3 cups unsalted turkey broth
2/3 cup skim milk (replaces 2/3 cup of table cream)
1 1/2 cups cook, diced turkey

1. For pastry, mix flour and salt thoroughly.
2. Mix 3 tablespoons flour mixture with water to make a paste.
3. Using a fork, lightly mix oil with remaining flour mixture until mixture is crumbly.
4. Stir flour paste into flour-oil mixture to form a ball. Divide into 4 pieces.

5. Roll each piece between 2 sheets of wax paper until the dough is at least 1/2-inch wider all around than baking dishes.

6. For filling, add vegetables to boiling water. Cover and boil gently until vegetables are just tender, about 6 minutes. Drain.

7. Melt margarine; stir in flour and seasonings.

8. Add broth and milk slowly, stirring constantly; cook until thickened.

9. Stir in turkey and vegetables.

10. Pour into 4 1-cup baking dishes.

11. Remove top paper from each piece of rolled pastry. Invert pastry, paper side up, over each dish of filling. Peel off remaining papers. Fold edges under to rim of dishes.

12. Flute edges of dough with fingers or press lightly with tines of fork. Cut several small slits in dough for steam to escape during baking.

13. Bake at 400°F (hot oven) until crusts are browned and filling is bubbly, about 40 minutes.

Mixes Made Slim

Packaged mixes don't usually win rave reviews from nutrition-ists when it comes to fat content. But you can trim some of the fat from macaroni and cheese, brownies, and scalloped pota-toes. Do your deducting from the ingredients-to-add column, which is where most of the fat typically comes from anyway.

If you use casserole or noodle mixes that call for hamburger, try substituting lean ground turkey or extra-lean ground beef. With macaroni and cheese packets, stir in only half the margarine called for, and switch to skim milk instead of whole. Ditto for scalloped potatoes, instant rice, and pasta salads. Changes won't affect flavor significantly, and the product becomes lower in fat.

Make fat deductions carefully with bakery mixes like muffins, pancakes, and quick breads. Fat influences the texture of baked goods. You can pull off little switches like using two egg whites for each egg and skim milk in place of whole. But decreasing oil and shortening yields mixed results. After a bit of trial and error, you may hit on a successful adjustment.

Another option: It's possible to replace fat entirely or almost entirely in products like cake or brownie mixes with moist ingredients like applesauce and plain, nonfat yogurt. Substitute 1/2 cup of plain, nonfat yogurt for oil and eggs in your favorite brownie mix. Pans must still be greased, but no extra fat is added.

If you have questions about making substitutions with mixes, check the package to see if a toll-free number is listed for prod-uct information. You can call and find out what lower-fat options work with various mixes.

Substitutions

Here's a summary of other fat-saving substitutions you might like to try.

Evaporated skim milk: For a rich, creamy sauce or soup that's low in fat and calories, use evaporated skim milk instead of heavy cream. It has a cream-like flavor and is richer in texture than regular skim milk. Best of all, you'll slim down your recipe by more than 80 grams of fat and 600 calories for every cup used.

Fat-free plain yogurt: Use fat-free plain yogurt in place of sour cream. Try this in your stroganoff recipe and even in ambrosia salad.

Applesauce: Rather than using oil, margarine, or butter in many baked products, substitute applesauce. This substitution works well in muffins, quick breads, cake mixes, and cakes made from scratch. Applesauce is rich in a natural substance called pectin, which, like fat, prevents moisture loss during baking.

In recipes, where oil is the only liquid, use a combination of half applesauce and half low-fat buttermilk. Buttermilk is a good choice because it has more body than other liquids, such as skim milk, fruit juice, or water.

Prunes: Pureed prunes or baby food prunes are one of the best fat replacers in chocolate baked goodies, such as brownies and cakes. They add a naturally sweet flavor and chewy texture. For ease and convenience, try baby food prunes instead of pureeing your own. To puree prunes, place 2/3 cup or 4 ounces of pitted prunes in a blender or small food processor. Add 3 tablespoons of hot water and blend or process until the prunes are smooth.

Marshmallow creme: If you want a fluffy frosting, replace the margarine or butter in your recipe with marshmallow creme. It adds a creaminess to the frosting without contributing any fat.

Reduced-calorie margarine or butter: If a recipe calls for a solid fat—like shortening, butter, or margarine—try replacing it with reduced-calorie margarine or butter. These products are made lighter by having water whipped into them. But remember, even though one tablespoon of a reduced calorie product is lower in calories and fat than its regular counterpart, all of those calories still come from fat.

Generally it's best to use these products in foods that won't be cooked. In some recipes, such as cookies, the additional water from the margarine or butter will change the texture of the product.

Fruit juice: For a nonfat salad dressing or marinade, use fruit juice. White grape, apple, orange, and pineapple juices are all light-flavored alternatives to oil. Or combine the juice with defatted chicken broth for a less fruity liquid.

Egg whites: For each whole egg, use two egg whites. Although you'll only save 5 grams of fat, the bigger savings will be in cholesterol. One egg yolk contains 213 milligrams of cholesterol.

Cocoa powder: For great chocolate flavor without the fat, use cocoa powder. For each ounce of unsweetened chocolate, use 3 tablespoons unsweetened cocoa powder. Adding a small amount of instant coffee granules, about 1/2 to 1 teaspoon per recipe, enhances the chocolate flavor.

Cream soup: Make your own low-fat cream soup to replace those you once bought in cans and used in casseroles. In a small saucepan, use a wire whisk to stir together 1 cup of evaporated skim milk, 1 tablespoon cornstarch, and 1 teaspoon instant low-sodium bouillon granules. Cook and stir until thickened and bubbly. Cook and stir for 1 minute more.

What Are You Saving?

Skim away fat and calories from recipes by trying some of these easy-to-adjust-to substitutions. Before long your meals will be well within healthful fat limits.

Instead of . . .	substitute . . .			and save
		Fat (gm.)	Cholesterol (mg.)	Calories
Whole milk	Skim milk	8	30	64 per cup
Whole egg, 1	Egg whites, 2	6	213	47
Cream cheese	Neufchatel cheese	3	6	24 per ounce
Ricotta cheese	1% cottage cheese	14	53	52 per 1/2 cup
Cheddar cheese	Mozzarella, skim	4	12	42 per ounce
Heavy cream	Half and half	32	3	15 per tablespoon
Sour cream	Low-fat yogurt	18	33	172 per 1/2 cup
Fudge sauce	Chocolate syrup	4	0	32 per 2 tablespoons

Skimming Your Favorite Recipes

Here are some more ways to save your favorite recipes:

1. Reduce the amount of fat called for. If the fat ingredient is a necessary part of the final product, you may not be able to totally eliminate it. Oil in pesto sauce, for example, is essential

or you won't have pesto sauce, but you can usually decrease the amount of fat needed.

2. Remove the fat ingredient entirely when possible. When you look at the recipe, ask yourself whether the fatty ingredient is there for appearance or simply as a tradition. If it's the latter, eliminate it altogether.

3. Use something else lower in fat to replace the fatty ingredient. Is the ingredient there for flavor or texture? Can you get almost the same effect by adding another lower-fat item, like low-fat yogurt or 1% cottage cheese?

4. When you can, use the substitutions listed above, or try the ones listed below:

Instead of butter, shortening, or margarine, use:

—Powdered butter substitutes (except for stir-fry dishes)

—Butter-flavored sprinkles over foods like baked potatoes and popcorn

—Margarine with liquid vegetable oil listed first on its ingredient list. Use less than is called for, even up to half less.

—Liquids like wine, fruit juice, or chicken broth whenever the recipe is using a fatty ingredient to add moisture.

▲ Instead of baking chocolate, which is very high in fat, use 3 tablespoons cocoa powder and 1 tablespoon oil.

▲ Instead of hot chocolate mixes, use hot cocoa mix made from 1 cup nonfat, dry milk powder, 1/3 cup unsweetened cocoa powder, and 3 tablespoons sugar. Mix these ingredients in an airtight container. To use, put 2 heaping teaspoons of mix into a cup and add hot water. Stir well and enjoy.

▲ Instead of full-fat cheeses, use part-skim mozzarella and other reduced fat cheeses. Use less cheese than the recipe calls for to save more fat and calories.

▲ Instead of whole milk ricotta cheese, use part-skim ricotta cheese or 1% fat cottage cheese, or a mixture of the two.

▲ Instead of cream, use evaporated skim milk or regular nonfat milk. Add some nonfat dry milk to thicken if needed. Nondairy creamers may be labeled no cholesterol, but they can be very high in fat, so be careful.

▲ Instead of regular cream cheese, use Neufchatel cheese or a light (reduced-fat) cream cheese, or combine these with plain nonfat yogurt, part-skim ricotta, or low-fat cottage cheese.

▲ Instead of creamy dressings or dips, use this creamy dressing that is nearly fat free:

—1 small envelope (1 oz.) ranch dressing powder (reduced calorie)

—1 1/2 cups nonfat milk

—1/2 cup nonfat plain yogurt

—1 tablespoon "light" mayonnaise (reduced fat and calorie)

Blend the milk, yogurt, mayo, and powder together well. Keeps in the refrigerator for about five days. Makes two cups.

▲ Instead of eggs, use egg whites or egg substitutes. Three eggs can be replaced by one egg beaten with three egg whites.

▲ Instead of mayonnaise, use plain yogurt, reduced-calorie mayonnaise, or low-fat cottage cheese, or make your own mock mayonnaise by mixing 1/2 cup reduced calorie, low fat mayonnaise with 1/2 cup low-fat plain yogurt.

▲ Instead of sour cream, use nonfat or low-fat plain yogurt. In sauces, add 2 tablespoons of flour for each cup of yogurt so the sauce will thicken properly. In hot dishes, stir the yogurt in just before serving, since high temperatures cause it to curdle.

▲ Or try light sour cream, or substitute part-skim ricotta cheese or low-fat cottage cheese blended with buttermilk. But be wary, most imitation sour creams have just as much fat as regular sour cream.

▲ Instead of some or all of the fat for stir-frying, simmering, or sauteing, use low-sodium broths, wine, beer, or fruit juice.

▲ Replace some of the fat in certain recipes with fruit juices, fruit purees, or buttermilk or small amounts of rum, whiskey, or brandy.

Flavor With No Fat

Flavor is the main appeal for much of the food we prefer to eat, and often it is the fat that gives the flavor. When you want to get rid of the fat, but keep the flavor, here are some more possible substitutions:

Flavored extracts to have on hand

Almond, mint, lemon, rum, vanilla, coconut, butter, orange, liquid smoke

Other liquids

Low-sodium soy sauce, flavored vinegars

Vegetable flavorings

Ginger root, onions, celery, garlic shallots, horseradish

Fruits

Lemons, lemon peel, oranges, orange peel, limes, grapefruit, fruit purees (berries, melons, peaches, prunes, dried apricots)

Must-have herbs and spices

Basil, dill, tarragon, oregano, cumin, coriander, freshly ground pepper, thyme, sage, garlic powder

Highly flavored sweeteners

Molasses, brown sugar, maple syrup, concentrated fruit juices

Liquor and liqueurs

Orange or coffee flavored liqueurs, amaretto, vermouth, sherry, wine, beer, creme de menthe

Fat replacements for cooking on the stove:

low sodium chicken, beef, or vegetable broth
fruit juices
garlic wine
flavored vinegars
plain water
low-fat milk or evaporated skim milk
nonfat sour cream
wine
regular or nonalcoholic beer
other liquor like brandy, vermouth

Fat replacements for the oven:

nonfat or light cream cheese
nonfat or light sour cream
nonfat or low-fat flavored yogurts
fruit juice and fruit purees
evaporated skim milk
liquor and liqueurs

Summary Guidelines
for Replacing Fat in Recipes

Remember, when you take fat out of a recipe, you often need to add some liquid ingredient (preferably one with no or low fat) to make up the difference in liquid volume and moistening power. So with the fat replacement program in place, you can often bring down the chief fat ingredient to low levels and still have a food that looks and tastes like the original. Here are more examples:

▲ In muffins and nut breads, bring down the oil, butter, or margarine to 2 tablespoons per 12-muffin recipe.

▲ In homemade cakes and coffee cakes, you can reduce the fat to 1/4 to 1/3 cup per cake.

▲ In cake mixes, you can eliminate the fat altogether by substituting something compatible with the flavor of the cake. Try nonfat sour cream, applesauce, pineapple juice, flavored yogurt, evaporated skim milk, or pureed baby fruits.

▲ In biscuits, reduce the fat from 1/2 cup to 4 tablespoons per every 2 cups of flour, but remember to add some fat replacement to make up the volume. Try nonfat sour cream or light cream cheese.

▲ In pie crust, reduce the fat to 3 tablespoons for every cup of flour, and increase the water to about 3 tablespoons for every cup of flour.

▲ In cookies, cut the fat in half, then add a substitute.

▲ In cheese sauce, eliminate any butter or margarine altogether. Make a thickening paste by mixing flour with a little bit of milk, add the cheese, and whisk in more milk to get the consistency you want.

▲ In tomato sauces, simply eliminate the oil altogether. Use herbs and spices if you want to vary the flavor.

▲ In marinades, the most important ingredient is the acidic liquid that tenderizes the meat, not the fat. So use wine, beer, tomato juice, or vinegar in marinade recipes, and eliminate the fat altogether. Add the flavoring, herbs, and spices you like to retain the taste.

▲ In vinaigrette dressings, instead of the traditional three parts oil and one part vinegar, switch to three parts vinegar and one part oil. Use rice vinegar for a milder flavor.

▲ For pan frying or sauteing, eliminate the fat and use vegetable broth, wine, or water.

Main Dishes

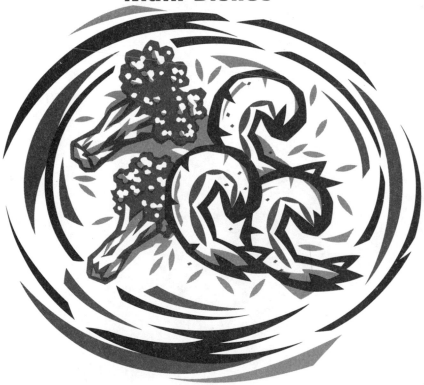

Skim the Fat

Southwestern Pork

1 1/2 pound pork tenderloin
2 teaspoons ground cumin
1/4 cup cornmeal
2 teaspoons vegetable oil
1 cup reduced-sodium chicken broth
2 tablespoons red wine vinegar
3 tablespoons tomato paste
1 tablespoon brown sugar
2 stalks celery, sliced on the diagonal
2 carrots, peeled and sliced on the diagonal
1/2 cup frozen kernel corn
1/2 red pepper, sliced into thin, short strips

1. Trim excess fat from tenderloin; cut into 2 sections if not already in 2 pieces.
2. Mix cumin with cornmeal. Roll tenderloin sections in mixture to coat.
3. Pour oil into a nonstick, 12-inch skillet, and turn heat to medium.
4. Add tenderloin, and allow it to brown evenly on all sides.
5. Mix chicken broth, vinegar, tomato paste, and sugar together. Add to pan with celery and carrots.
6. Bring mixture to a boil; cover and simmer 15 to 20 minutes.
7. Add corn and red pepper; cover and simmer 10 more minutes.
8. To serve, slice meat onto a platter and surround with vegetables.

8 SERVINGS
170 CALORIES PER SERVING;
4.9 GRAMS OF FAT; 1.3 GRAMS OF SATURATED FAT;
60 MILLIGRAMS OF CHOLESTEROL

Hungarian Meatloaf

8-ounce package chopped coleslaw mix,
or 1/2 cup shredded cabbage
2 egg whites
1 tablespoon paprika
1 tablespoon thyme
2 teaspoons cayenne pepper
2 slices white bread
1 1/4 pound lean (7% fat) ground turkey
Vegetable cooking spray

....

1. Place coleslaw mix or cabbage in a small mixing bowl. Stir in egg whites and seasonings.

2. Crumble bread and add bread crumbs with turkey to mixing bowl. Mix gently.

3. Lightly coat a 9-inch loaf pan with vegetable cooking spray. Place turkey mixture into pan.

4. Bake at 350°F for 45 to 50 minutes.

....

8 SERVINGS
120 CALORIES PER SERVING;
5.8 GRAMS OF FAT; 1.5 GRAMS OF SATURATED FAT;
25 MILLIGRAMS OF CHOLESTEROL

Turkey and Wild Rice Casserole

1/2 cup natural long-grain and wild rice (about 3 ounces)
2 cups water
1/4 teaspoon salt
8 ounces fresh mushrooms, sliced
1 tablespoon margarine
2 tablespoons flour
1 cup skim milk
1 teaspoon chicken bouillon granules
1/16 teaspoon pepper
2 cups cubed, cooked turkey (about 12 ounces)
4 tablespoons sliced pimento
1/2 cup sliced water chestnuts (about 2 ounces)
1/4 cup sliced almonds (about 1 ounce)

1. Wash rice. Add water and salt, bring to boil, cover, and simmer about 1 hour until water is absorbed.

2. In large skillet, saute mushrooms in margarine about 3 minutes. Stir in flour. Add milk, bouillon, and pepper. Cook until thickened, stirring constantly.

3. Add turkey, pimento, water chestnuts, and rice. Mix and pour into a 7- by 11-inch baking dish. Sprinkle with sliced almonds.

4. Cover and bake in 350°F oven for 30 minutes. Uncover and bake about 3 more minutes. Cut into 6 servings, 2 inches by 3 inches.

6 SERVINGS
233 CALORIES; 7.7 GRAMS OF FAT;
2 GRAMS OF SATURATED FAT; 45 MILLIGRAMS OF CHOLESTEROL

Shrimp and Broccoli Saute

1/4 cup reduced-sodium soy sauce
1/4 cup chicken broth, defatted
2 tablespoons water
2 teaspoons cornstarch
1 teaspoon packed brown sugar
1 tablespoon vegetable oil
1 piece (1 1/2 inches) peeled fresh ginger,
cut into 1/4-inch thick slices
2 large garlic cloves, halved
1 medium onion, sliced thin
1 pound shrimp, peeled and deveined
1/8 to 1/4 teaspoon crushed red pepper
4 cups small broccoli florets, cooked
1 cup long-grain rice, cooked

1. Combine soy sauce, chicken broth, water, cornstarch, and brown sugar in bowl.

2. Heat oil in large nonstick skillet over medium-high heat. Add ginger and garlic; cook, stirring, until garlic is just golden. Discard ginger and garlic. Add onion to skillet. Cook, stirring frequently until tender, about 5 minutes.

3. Add shrimp and pepper to skillet; toss. Stir in soy mixture. Cover and simmer, stirring once, until shrimp are opaque, about 3 to 4 minutes. Stir in broccoli and heat through. Serve with rice.

4 SERVINGS
360 CALORIES PER SERVING
6 GRAMS OF FAT; 1 GRAM OF SATURATED FAT
140 MILLIGRAMS OF CHOLESTEROL

Cajun Black Beans and Rice

2 Italian turkey sausage links
2 teaspoons vegetable oil
1 large onion, chopped
1 green pepper, diced
2 cloves garlic, crushed
1 tablespoon cajun spices
3 tablespoons red wine vinegar
2 tablespoons water
3 cups black beans, cooked (1 cup uncooked)
2 cups rice, cooked (about 2/3 cup uncooked)
1 red pepper, diced

1. Cook sausage according to package directions. Drain and crumble into pieces with a fork; set aside.

2. Place oil in a nonstick skillet; add onion, green pepper, and garlic. Turn heat to low and saute uncovered for 10 minutes or until tender.

3. Return sausage to skillet; add cajun spices, vinegar, and water and stir.

4. Add precooked beans; cover and simmer over low heat for 5 to 10 minutes to allow flavors to blend.

5. Divide cooked rice among six soup bowls. Ladle beans over rice and top with diced red pepper.

6 SERVINGS, ABOUT 1 CUP EACH
310 CALORIES PER SERVING; 8 GRAMS OF FAT;
2.4 GRAMS OF SATURATED FAT; 15 MILLIGRAMS OF CHOLESTEROL

Vegetable Beef Stir-Fry

1 pound boneless top round steak, partially frozen
2 tablespoons reduced-sodium soy sauce
1 tablespoon garlic, finely chopped
2 teaspoons sesame oil
1 red pepper, julienned
1 yellow pepper, julienned
1 carrot, julienned
1/2 pound snow peas
5 tablespoons water
4 1/2 cups brown rice, cooked (about 1 1/2 cups uncooked)

Sauce:
3/4 teaspoon cornstarch
2 tablespoons reduced-sodium soy sauce
1 1/2 tablespoons dry sherry
1 tablespoon honey

1. Slice meat across the grain and on the diagonal to make thin strips.

2. Pour soy sauce and garlic into a bowl; add meat strips and toss gently to coat. Set aside.

3. Heat the oil in a large wok or frying pan (use high heat for stir-frying) and add peppers and carrot. Stir a minute or two, and then add snow peas and water.

4. Cook for another 2 to 3 minutes, stirring occasionally until vegetables are tender but crisp.

5. Remove vegetables from wok and add meat and its liquid to wok. Cook for about 5 to 8 minutes, stirring frequently.

6. Return vegetables to wok.

7. Mix sauce ingredients together and add to wok; stir until sauce boils and thickens.

8. Serve over hot rice.

6 SERVINGS, 3/4 CUP RICE AND 1 CUP STIR-FRY EACH
335 CALORIES PER SERVING; 7.7 GRAMS OF FAT;
2.4 GRAMS OF SATURATED FAT; 45 MILLIGRAMS OF CHOLESTEROL

Navy Beans and Ham

1 cup dry pea (navy) beans
4 cups boiling water
1/2 cup onion, sliced
1 cup lean ham, cooked and diced
1/4 teaspoon salt
1 bay leaf
1/8 teaspoon pepper
1 cup carrots, sliced
1/4 cup celery, diced
2 teaspoons flour
1 tablespoon water

1. Add beans to boiling water. Return to boiling and boil 2 minutes. Remove from heat, cover, and soak 1 hour.

2. Return beans and water to boiling; add onion, ham, and seasonings. Boil uncovered for 5 minutes, then cover and boil gently until beans are almost tender (about 1 hour).

3. Add carrots and celery. Cook until tender (about 20 minutes). Remove bay leaf.

4. Mix flour with 1 tablespoon of water until smooth. Add slowly to beans, stirring constantly; cook until thickened.

4 SERVINGS, ABOUT 1 CUP EACH
165 CALORIES PER SERVING; 2.4 GRAMS OF FAT;
0.8 GRAM OF SATURATED FAT; 20 MILLIGRAMS OF CHOLESTEROL

Chicken Curry

1/4 cup onion, chopped
2 cups tart apple, cored and chopped
1 tablespoon oil
2 tablespoons flour
1/2 teaspoon salt
1/8 teaspoon ground ginger
1 teaspoon curry powder
1 cup skim milk
1 1/2 cups chicken, cooked and diced
1/4 cup raisins
2 cups brown rice, cooked (about 2/3 cup uncooked)

1. Cook onion and apple in oil until tender.

2. Stir in flour, salt, ginger, and curry powder. Add milk slowly, stirring constantly; cook until thickened.

3. Add chicken and raisins. Heat to serving temperature. Serve over rice.

4 SERVINGS, ABOUT 2/3 CUP CURRY
AND 1/2 CUP RICE EACH
330 CALORIES PER SERVING; 7.1 GRAMS OF FAT;
1.4 GRAMS OF SATURATED FAT; 45 MILLIGRAMS OF CHOLESTEROL

Mexican Macaroni

1/2 cup onion, chopped
1/4 cup green pepper, chopped
1/4 cup celery, chopped
3/4 pound ground beef, extra lean
16-ounce can tomatoes
10 3/4-ounce can tomato puree
1 teaspoon chili powder
1/4 teaspoon salt
1/8 teaspoon pepper
3 cups elbow macaroni, cooked and unsalted
(about 1 cup uncooked)

1. Saute onion, green pepper, and celery in a large nonstick frying pan until onion is clear. Remove from pan. Add beef and cook until beef is lightly browned. Drain.

2. Break up large pieces of tomatoes. Add tomatoes, tomato puree, vegetables, and seasonings to beef mixture. Simmer 15 minutes to blend flavors.

3. Stir in macaroni. Heat to serving temperature.

Menu suggestion: Serve with hot French bread.

4 SERVINGS, ABOUT 1 1/3 CUP EACH
380 CALORIES PER SERVING; 11.4 GRAMS OF FAT;
4.2 GRAMS OF SATURATED FAT; 55 MILLIGRAMS OF CHOLESTEROL

Turkey Tetrazzini

Vegetable cooking spray
2-ounce can mushroom stems and pieces
2 tablespoons green pepper, chopped
2 tablespoons oil
3 tablespoons flour
1/2 teaspoon salt
Dash of pepper
1/2 cup turkey or chicken broth
13-ounce can evaporated skim milk
2 tablespoons sherry (optional)
1 1/2 cups turkey, cooked and diced
1 tablespoon pimento, chopped
2 cups thin spaghetti, cooked and unsalted
(about 4 ounces uncooked)
1 tablespoon grated Parmesan cheese

1. Grease a 1 1/2-quart casserole with vegetable cooking spray.
2. Cook mushrooms and green pepper in oil until green pepper is tender. Stir in flour, salt, and pepper.
3. Mix broth with milk. Add slowly to flour mixture, stirring constantly; cook until thickened. Stir in sherry (optional), turkey, and pimento.
4. Mix in spaghetti and pour into casserole. Sprinkle with cheese. Bake at 350°F until bubbly throughout (about 30 minutes).

4 SERVINGS, ABOUT 1 CUP EACH
350 CALORIES PER SERVING; 10 GRAMS OF FAT;
1.9 GRAMS OF SATURATED FAT; 40 MILLIGRAMS OF CHOLESTEROL

Italian Fish Roll-Ups

1 pound flounder or cod fillets, fresh or frozen, without skin
9-ounce package frozen, French-style green beans
2 tablespoons onion, chopped
1/2 cup boiling water
8-ounce can tomato sauce
1/4 teaspoon dried oregano
1/4 teaspoon dried basil
1/8 teaspoon garlic powder
1 tablespoon Parmesan cheese, grated

1. Thaw frozen fish in refrigerator overnight. Divide fish into 4 servings.

2. Add beans and onion to boiling water. Cover and boil gently until beans are tender-crisp, about 7 minutes. Drain.

3. Place 1/4 of the bean-onion mixture in the middle of each fish portion.

4. Start with the narrow end of each fillet and roll. Place in a baking pan with the end of fillets underneath.

5. Mix tomato sauce, oregano, basil, and garlic powder. Pour over fish roll-ups.

6. Sprinkle with cheese.

7. Bake at 350°F until fish flakes easily when tested with a fork, about 45 minutes.

4 SERVINGS, 1 ROLL UP EACH
125 CALORIES PER SERVING;
1.5 GRAMS OF FAT; 0.5 GRAM OF SATURATED FAT;
49 MILLIGRAMS OF CHOLESTEROL

Skim the Fat

Meatless Main Dishes

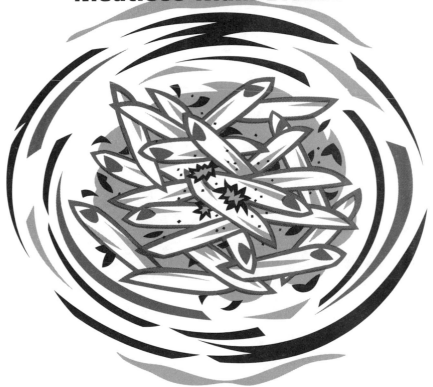

Skim the Fat

Pasta Primavera

6 cups water
8 ounces thin spaghetti, broken into 2-inch lengths
2 tablespoons margarine
1 cup onion, cut into thin wedges
2 cups broccoli, cut into florets and stalks peeled and sliced
1 cup carrots, thinly sliced
1 cup zucchini, thinly sliced
1 cup yellow summer squash, diced
3/4 cup water
3/4 teaspoon chicken bouillon granules
6 tablespoons parsley, chopped
3 tablespoons lemon juice
1 1/2 teaspoons basil
1/4 teaspoon pepper
3 tablespoons grated Parmesan cheese

1. Bring water to a boil, add spaghetti, stir, and boil gently until tender, about 10 minutes. Meanwhile, prepare vegetables.

2. Heat margarine in a large skillet. Add onion. Stir-fry about 1 minute.

3. Add vegetables. Stir. Add water and chicken bouillon. Stir. Cover and simmer about 6 minutes.

4. Add parsley, lemon juice, basil, and pepper. Stir and cook 1 minute.

5. Drain spaghetti and add to vegetables.

6. Sprinkle with Parmesan cheese; toss to mix well.

6 SERVINGS, 1 1/2 CUP PER SERVING
222 CALORIES; 5.5 GRAMS FAT; 1 GRAM OF SATURATED FAT;
2 MILLIGRAMS CHOLESTEROL

Two-Bean Chili

1 large onion, coarsely chopped (2 cups)
2 cloves garlic, minced
2 teaspoons oil
14 1/2-ounce can no-salt-added stewed tomatoes
1 can or bottle beer (12 ounces)
1 tablespoon chili powder
1 teaspoon ground cumin
1 teaspoon hot pepper sauce or hot salsa or picante sauce
1/4 teaspoon salt (optional)
15-ounce can pinto beans, rinsed and drained
1 can (about 16 ounces) dark red kidney beans,
rinsed and drained
1 large green bell pepper, coarsely chopped (2 cups, 8 ounces)
1/4 cup chopped cilantro

1. Saute onion and garlic in large saucepan or Dutch oven in oil until tender, about 4 minutes. Stir in tomatoes, beer, chili powder, cumin, hot sauce, and salt, if desired.

2. Simmer uncovered 15 minutes. Stir in beans and green pepper. Simmer uncovered 15 minutes. Sprinkle with cilantro.

Microwave Method

1. Toss onion and garlic with oil in 2 1/2-quart microwave-safe casserole dish. Cover and cook on high power 3 minutes. Stir in tomatoes, beer, chili powder, cumin, hot sauce, and salt, if desired.

2. Cover and cook on high power until boiling, 5 to 6 minutes. Stir; reduce power to medium and cook 12 minutes, stirring once. Add beans and bell pepper.

3. Microwave version of chili will be thinner. If desired, combine 2 tablespoons cornstarch and 2 tablespoons water. Stir into chili; cover and cook on high power 2 minutes.

7 SERVINGS, 1 CUP EACH; 174 CALORIES; 2.1 GRAMS OF FAT;
TRACE OF SATURATED FAT; 0 CHOLESTEROL

Green-Pea Curry with Rice

1 1/2 cups green split peas (about 12 ounces)
3 cups water
1 1/2 teaspoons vegetable oil
1 cup chopped onion
1 tablespoon curry powder
3/4 teaspoon ground ginger
3 tablespoons raisins
1/4 teaspoon salt (optional)
1 cup water
3 cups cooked rice

1. Wash peas, add water, bring to boil. Cover, remove from heat, and let stand 1 hour.
2. Heat oil in saucepan. Add onions and saute until limp. Add spices and raisins. Stir to blend.
3. Add green peas and water as needed to cover. Stir. Bring to a boil. Cover and simmer 1 hour.
4. Serve over 1/2 cup cooked rice.
5. Garnish with chutney, if desired.

Variation: One or a combination of the following may be used.

3/4 teaspoon cinnamon
3/4 teaspoon cumin
1 tablespoon toasted sesame seeds

6 SERVINGS, 3/4 CUP EACH
286 CALORIES PER SERVING;
1.9 GRAMS OF FAT; TRACE OF SATURATED FAT; 0 CHOLESTEROL

Baked Lentils au Gratin

Nonstick vegetable spray
1/4 cup onion, chopped
1/2 cup carrot, shredded
1 clove garlic, minced
2 cups cooked lentils (1 cup dry)
8-ounce can stewed tomatoes, undrained
1/4 small red bell pepper, chopped
1/2 teaspoon salt
1/8 teaspoon black pepper
1/8 teaspoon basil
1/8 teaspoon oregano, crushed
1/4 cup Monterey Jack cheese, shredded

....

1. Preheat oven to 375°F. Spray 2-quart casserole with nonstick vegetable spray.

2. Spray 8-inch skillet with nonstick vegetable spray. Saute onion, carrot, and garlic until soft. Pour into prepared casserole.

3. Add remaining ingredients except cheese.

4. Cover and bake for 45 minutes.

5. Uncover and sprinkle with cheese; bake for 5 to 7 minutes or until cheese is melted.

Microwave Method

1. Combine onion, carrot, and garlic in 2-quart microwave-safe casserole. Cover and cook for 5 minutes on high power, stirring once.

2. Stir in rest of ingredients except cheese. Cover and cook on medium-high power for 12 to 15 minutes, stirring once.

3. Uncover and top with cheese; cook for 50 seconds or until cheese melts.

....

4 SERVINGS, 3/4 CUP EACH
161 CALORIES PER SERVING; 2 GRAMS OF FAT;
1 GRAM OF SATURATED FAT; 7 MILLIGRAMS OF CHOLESTEROL

Soup and Salads

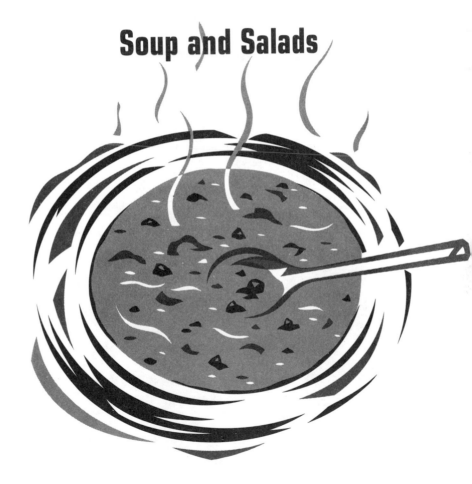

Creamy Fish Chowder

1 pound haddock fillets, fresh or frozen, without skin
1 1/2 cups potatoes, diced 1/4 inch thick
2 tablespoons onion, chopped
1 cup boiling water
2 tablespoons flour
2 tablespoons water
2 cups skim milk
1/2 teaspoon salt
Dash of pepper
1 tablespoon margarine

1. Thaw fish in refrigerator overnight. Cut into 1-inch pieces.
2. Add fish, potatoes, and onion to boiling water. Cover and simmer until potatoes are just tender (about 10 minutes). Drain.
3. Mix flour with 2 tablespoons of water until smooth. Stir into milk. Add milk mixture, salt, and pepper to fish mixture. Cook, stirring gently, until thickened. Stir in margarine.

4 SERVINGS, ABOUT 1 CUP EACH
200 CALORIES PER SERVING; 3.8 GRAMS OF FAT;
0.8 GRAM OF SATURATED FAT; 45 MILLIGRAMS OF CHOLESTEROL

Black Bean Soup

1 pound dried black beans
2 quarts water
3 teaspoons salt
2 tablespoons olive oil
2 cups chopped onions
1 cup chopped green pepper (optional)
2 teaspoons minced garlic
1 teaspoon ground cumin
1 teaspoon oregano
1/4 teaspoon dry mustard
1 tablespoon lemon juice

1. Presoak beans in water overnight or use quick-cook method on package.

2. After soaking beans, add 2 teaspoons salt and bring to a boil; cover and simmer on low heat for 2 hours.

3. Heat oil, add onions, and saute about 5 minutes. Add green pepper and saute until onions are tender.

4. Stir in remaining ingredients. Add about 3/4 cup hot bean liquid, cover, and simmer 10 minutes.

5. Add onion/seasoning mixture to beans and continue to cook 1 hour, stirring occasionally.

6. Serve over cooked brown rice, and top with chopped green onions. Freeze leftovers and reheat for another meal.

8 SERVINGS, 1 CUP EACH
241 CALORIES PER CUP, 4.4 GRAMS OF FAT;
1 GRAM OF SATURATED FAT; 0 CHOLESTEROL

Chunky Tarragon Chicken Salad

1 1/4 cup plain, nonfat yogurt
1 tablespoon Dijon mustard
1 tablespoon lemon rind, grated
2 teaspoons dried tarragon, crumbled
Black pepper, freshly ground, to taste
1 1/2 pound boneless, skinless chicken breast, poached or
microwaved
2 large celery stalks, chopped into thick pieces
1/2 cup red pepper, chopped
1 large, red Delicious apple, cored and chopped
1/4 cup almonds, sliced

....

1. Combine yogurt, mustard, lemon rind, tarragon, and pepper. Set aside.
2. Cut chicken into large chunks. Combine chicken, vegetables, apple, and almonds in bowl. Toss lightly.
3. Pour dressing over salad ingredients. Cover and refrigerate at least 2 hours to allow flavors to blend.

....

10 SERVINGS, 1/2 CUP EACH
167 CALORIES PER SERVING; 4.6 GRAMS OF FAT;
0.9 GRAM OF SATURATED FAT; 58 MILLIGRAMS OF CHOLESTEROL

Mock French Dressing

1 1/2 tablespoons cornstarch
2 tablespoons sugar
1 cup water
1/4 cup vinegar
1/4 teaspoon salt
1/2 teaspoon dry mustard
1/2 teaspoon paprika
1/8 teaspoon onion powder
Dash of garlic powder

1. Mix cornstarch and sugar in saucepan. Stir in water.
2. Cook over low heat, stirring constantly, until thickened.
3. Cool slightly.
4. Add remaining ingredients. Mix thoroughly.
5. Chill.

16 SERVINGS, 1 TABLESPOON EACH
10 CALORIES PER TABLESPOON; TRACE OF FAT;
TRACE OF SATURATED FAT; 0 CHOLESTEROL

Yogurt-Dill Dressing

8-ounce carton plain, nonfat yogurt
2 teaspoons onion, very finely chopped
1 teaspoon lemon juice
1/2 teaspoon dried dill weed
1/4 teaspoon dry mustard
1/8 teaspoon garlic powder

1. Mix all ingredients thoroughly.

2. Chill.

3. Serve over tossed green salad.

16 SERVINGS, 1 TABLESPOON EACH
10 CALORIES PER TABLESPOON; 0.2 GRAM OF FAT;
0.1 GRAM OF SATURATED FAT; 1 MILLIGRAM OF CHOLESTEROL

Warm Harvest Potato Salad

1 pound (6 to 8) new red potatoes
1 carrot, peeled and julienned
2 scallions, chopped
1 tablespoon Dijon mustard
1 tablespoon dry sherry
1 teaspoon olive oil
1/2 teaspoon dried dill

1. Scrub potatoes; leave skin on and cut into quarters.

2. Steam potatoes and carrot together in a small saucepan over low heat for 10 to 15 minutes or until tender. Drain and remove from heat. Keep saucepan covered.

3. Mix remaining ingredients in a small serving dish. Stir in hot potatoes and carrot. Serve while warm.

4 SERVINGS, 1 CUP EACH
135 CALORIES PER SERVING; 1.3 GRAMS OF FAT;
0.2 GRAM OF SATURATED FAT; 0 CHOLESTEROL

Curried Tuna and Pasta Salad

6 1/2-ounce can water-packed tuna, drained
1 medium red apple, cored and chopped
2 stalks celery, sliced on the diagonal
1 cup corkscrew pasta noodles, cooked
1/2 cup nonfat, plain yogurt
1 tablespoon spicy mustard
1 tablespoon curry powder

1. Place tuna, apple, celery, and pasta in a serving dish; toss together gently.

2. Mix yogurt, mustard, and curry powder to form a dressing; fold dressing into tuna mixture and serve or chill for later.

4 SERVINGS, 3/4 CUP EACH
140 CALORIES PER SERVING; 0.8 GRAM OF FAT;
0.2 GRAM OF SATURATED FAT; 10 MILLIGRAMS OF CHOLESTEROL

Skim the Fat

Vegetables

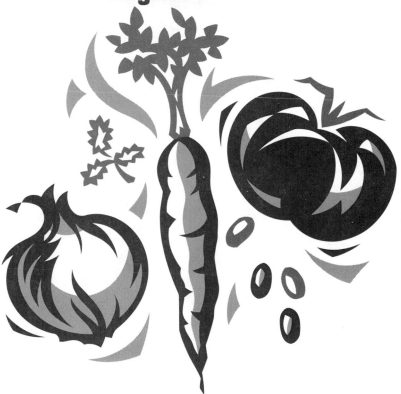

Skim the Fat

Roasted Zucchini

Vegetable cooking spray
4 small zucchini (about 1 pound total)
1 teaspoon olive oil
1 teaspoon balsamic vinegar
1 teaspoon dried basil
1/2 teaspoon black pepper
1 clove garlic, finely chopped

1. Lightly coat a baking sheet with vegetable cooking spray.
2. Slice zucchini 1/2-inch thick; cut each slice into quarters. Place in a small mixing bowl.
3. Drizzle oil, vinegar, and spices over zucchini chunks. Add garlic and toss lightly.
4. Transfer zucchini to baking sheet and bake in a preheated 450°F oven for 8 to 10 minutes.

4 SERVINGS, 2/3 CUP EACH
30 CALORIES PER SERVING; 1.2 GRAMS OF FAT;
0.2 GRAMS OF SATURATED FAT; 0 CHOLESTEROL

Sweet Potato Stew

1/2 tablespoon margarine
2 cups fresh sweet potatoes, cooked and sliced
8-ounce can crushed pineapple in natural juice
1/4 teaspoon ground cinnamon
1/8 teaspoon salt

1. Heat margarine in a large frying pan. Add potato slices and pineapple. Sprinkle with cinnamon and salt.

2. Simmer uncovered until most of the juice has evaporated (about 10 to 15 minutes), turning potato slices several times.

4 SERVINGS, ABOUT 1/2 CUP EACH
135 CALORIES PER SERVING; 1.6 GRAMS OF FAT;
0.3 GRAM OF SATURATED FAT; 0 CHOLESTEROL

Cheese-Baked Potatoes

2 baking potatoes (about 8 ounces each)
1/2 cup low-fat cottage cheese
1/4 cup skim milk
1/4 teaspoon salt
1/8 teaspoon pepper
Paprika to taste

1. Wash potatoes well. Prick skins in several places. Bake at 425°F until tender (50 to 60 minutes).

2. Remove from oven; cut in half. Scoop out insides of potatoes, leaving skins intact; save skins. Mash potatoes thoroughly.

3. Add remaining ingredients except paprika, and beat until fluffy. Put mashed potato mixture into potato skins. Sprinkle paprika over the tops.

4. Bake at 425°F until heated through and tops are lightly browned (about 10 minutes).

4 SERVINGS, 1/2 POTATO EACH
140 CALORIES PER SERVING; 0.7 GRAM OF FAT;
0.4 GRAM OF SATURATED FAT; 5 MILLIGRAMS OF CHOLESTEROL

Asparagus With Dijon Sauce

3/4 pound fresh asparagus spears
1/4 cup reduced-sodium chicken broth
2 teaspoons Dijon mustard or tarragon Dijon mustard
1 tablespoon grated Romano or Asiago cheese

....

1. Break woody ends off asparagus; place in skillet.
2. Pour broth over asparagus; cover and steam over medium heat until crisp-tender, about 4 minutes.
3. Remove asparagus to warm serving plate with slotted spatula; keep warm.
4. Add mustard to skillet; increase heat to high and bring to a boil, stirring constantly.
5. Pour over asparagus; sprinkle with cheese.

Microwave Method

1. Break woody ends off asparagus; place in 2-quart rectangular microwave-safe dish.
2. Pour broth over asparagus; cover with vented plastic wrap and cook on high power 3 to 4 minutes or until crisp-tender.
3. Pour off liquid into 1-cup glass measure. Keep asparagus covered.
4. Whisk mustard into juices. Cook uncovered at high power until boiling, about 30 seconds.
5. Pour over asparagus; sprinkle with cheese.

....

4 SERVINGS
20 CALORIES PER SERVING; 0.7 GRAM OF FAT;
0.4 GRAMS OF SATURATED FAT; 1 MILLIGRAM OF CHOLESTEROL

Braised Endive

2 whole Belgian endive (8 ounces)
1/2 cup reduced-sodium chicken broth
1 teaspoon Dijon mustard
1 teaspoon honey
Freshly ground black pepper

1. Cut endive lengthwise in half.

2. Combine broth, mustard, and honey in saucepan large enough to hold endive in one layer. Bring to a boil. Add endive to broth, cut side down; reduce heat. Cover and simmer until tender, about 5 minutes, basting once with liquid in saucepan.

3. Transfer endive and broth to shallow dish. Serve with pepper.

Microwave Method

1. Cut endive lengthwise in half.

2. Whisk together broth, mustard, and honey in shallow microwave-safe dish large enough to hold endive in one layer. Add endive to broth, cut side down; cover and cook on high power, 3 minutes. Baste endive with juices in dish. Cover and continue to cook until tender, 3 to 4 minutes. Serve with pepper.

2 SERVINGS, 1 ENDIVE EACH
29 CALORIES PER SERVING; 0.6 GRAM OF FAT;
0.2 GRAM OF SATURATED FAT; 0 CHOLESTEROL

Recipes for Reducing Fat

Breads

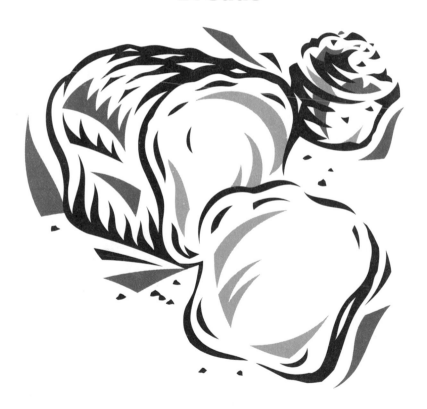

Skim the Fat

Honey Oatmeal Hotcakes

1 cup quick-cooking oats
1 cup skim milk
1 egg, beaten*
1 tablespoon honey
1 tablespoon vegetable oil
1/4 cup all-purpose flour
1/2 teaspoon baking powder
1/2 teaspoon baking soda
1/2 teaspoon cinnamon
Vegetable cooking spray
4 tablespoons marmalade (optional)

1. Combine oats and milk and let stand for 10 minutes.

2. Stir egg, honey, and oil into oat mixture.

3. In a separate bowl combine dry ingredients, including flour.

4. Add dry mixture to oats, stirring until moistened.

5. Pour 1/4 cup batter for each pancake onto a nonstick hot griddle or skillet that has been coated with cooking spray.

6. Turn pancakes when tops are covered with small bubbles and edges are firm.

7. (Optional) Spread 1/2 tablespoon of orange marmalade on pancakes while they are warm, or serve with pancake syrup.

4 SERVINGS, 2 4-INCH PANCAKES EACH
195 CALORIES PER SERVING; 6.1 GRAMS OF FAT;
1.1 GRAMS OF SATURATED FAT; 55 MILLIGRAMS OF CHOLESTEROL

*Substitute 2 egg whites for the egg if you want a cholesterol-free hotcake.

Herbed Breadsticks

1 *package active dry yeast*
1 *tablespoon brown sugar*
1 1/2 *cups warm water*
1 *teaspoon dry mustard*
2 *teaspoons dried rosemary*
2 *teaspoons dried oregano*
3 *cups whole wheat flour*
1 3/4 *cups all-purpose flour*
Flour for kneading
Vegetable cooking spray

....

1. Place yeast and sugar in a large mixing bowl, add warm water (about 110°F); let stand for 5 minutes.

2. Stir in mustard and spices. Add whole wheat flour and mix until moistened.

3. Gradually add the all-purpose flour, mixing until dough is no longer sticky.

4. Place dough onto a lightly floured surface, and knead for about 10 minutes or until smooth and elastic. Sprinkle on extra flour as needed.

5. Cut dough into 4 equal pieces; divide each piece into 6. On floured surface, roll each piece into a rope about 10 inches long.

6. Place ropes about 2 inches apart on a large, nonstick cookie sheet coated with vegetable cooking spray; leave uncovered.

7. Let ropes rise in a warm spot until they puff up slightly (about 20 minutes).

8. Bake at 400°F for 15 minutes.

....

24 BREADSTICKS
90 CALORIES PER BREADSTICK; 0.4 GRAM OF FAT;
0.1 GRAM OF SATURATED FAT; 0 CHOLESTEROL

Zucchini Muffins

Vegetable oil
2 cups whole wheat flour
1 tablespoon baking powder
1/2 teaspoon salt
1 teaspoon ground cinnamon
3/4 cup skim milk
2 egg whites, slightly beaten
1/4 cup oil
1/4 cup honey
1 cup zucchini squash, shredded

1. Preheat oven to 375°F and grease muffin tins lightly with oil.
2. Mix dry ingredients thoroughly. Mix remaining ingredients and add to dry ingredients. Stir until dry ingredients are barely moistened. Batter will be lumpy.
3. Fill muffin cups two-thirds full. Bake until lightly browned (about 20 minutes).

12 MUFFINS
140 CALORIES PER MUFFIN; 5 GRAMS OF FAT;
0.7 GRAM OF SATURATED FAT; TRACE OF CHOLESTEROL

Cranberry Bread

Vegetable oil
2 cups flour
1/2 cup sugar
1/2 teaspoon baking soda
1/2 teaspoon salt
Juice and rind of 1 medium orange
2 teaspoons melted margarine
Hot water
1 egg, beaten
1 teaspoon vanilla
1 cup cranberries, halved
1/2 cup chopped walnuts

1. Preheat oven to 350°F.
2. Cut aluminum foil to fit the bottom of a 9- by 5-inch loaf pan. Lightly grease sides of pan with vegetable oil.
3. Sift dry ingredients together.
4. Measure together orange juice, grated rind, and melted margarine; add enough hot water to make 1 cup.
5. Stir liquid into dry ingredients. Add remaining ingredients.
6. Add batter to prepared loaf pan. Bake for 1 hour or until toothpick inserted in top of loaf comes out clean.
7. Let stand overnight for easy slicing.

18 SERVINGS, 1/2-INCH SLICE EACH
110 CALORIES PER SERVING; 2.9 GRAMS OF FAT;
TRACE OF SATURATED FAT; 15 MILLIGRAMS OF CHOLESTEROL

Cheese and Basil Scones

2 cups flour
1/4 cup (1 ounce) freshly grated Parmesan
or Romano cheese
2 teaspoons baking powder
1/2 teaspoon baking soda
2 tablespoons chopped fresh basil leaves
or 2 teaspoons dried basil
1/4 teaspoon freshly ground black pepper
2/3 cup low-fat buttermilk
3 tablespoons good-quality olive oil
Nonstick vegetable spray
1 tablespoon egg substitute or 1 egg, beaten (optional)

1. Preheat oven to 450°F.
2. Combine flour, cheese, baking powder, soda, basil, and pepper in medium bowl.
3. Add buttermilk and oil; mix only until dry ingredients are moistened. Divide dough into 2 balls. Knead gently 3 times on floured surface.
4. Spray cookie sheet with vegetable spray. Pat dough into 2 circles, 7 to 8 inches in diameter. With sharp knife, score each circle (1/4 inch deep) into 6 wedges. Do not cut through.
5. Brush with egg or egg substitute, if desired, to glaze. Bake 10 to 12 minutes or until golden brown. Cut into wedges and serve warm or at room temperature.

12 SCONES
126 CALORIES PER SCONE; 4.1 GRAMS OF FAT;
0.7 GRAM OF SATURATED FAT; 2 MILLIGRAMS OF CHOLESTEROL

Note: Scones may be wrapped securely and frozen for up to 3 months. Reheat in 350°F oven uncovered 10 minutes, or wrap each scone in a paper towel and cook on high power in microwave oven for 30 to 40 seconds.

Skim the Fat

Desserts

Skim the Fat

Spicy Poached Pears

1 cup apple juice
1/2 cup cranberry juice cocktail
1 tablespoon orange juice
1/3 cup water
1/4 teaspoon ground cloves
1/4 teaspoon cinnamon
1/8 teaspoon ground ginger
4 ripe bosc pears, peeled

....

1. Pour juice, water, and spices into a deep saucepan; cover and bring to a boil.

2. Trim the bottom off pears, if necessary, so they stand up straight. Remove core.

3. Add pears and simmer uncovered until tender (15 to 25 minutes, depending on how ripe the pears are).

4. Remove pears and set aside.

5. Cook the remaining liquids over medium-high heat, stirring periodically, until mixture has reduced by half. Drizzle this juice-syrup over pears, and serve while warm, or chill and serve later.

....

4 SERVINGS
165 CALORIES PER SERVING; 0.7 GRAM OF FAT;
0.1 GRAM OF SATURATED FAT; 0 CHOLESTEROL

Dutch Gingerbread Cake

1 3/4 cups all-purpose flour
1 1/4 teaspoons baking soda
1 3/4 teaspoons ground ginger
1/2 teaspoon ground cloves
1/2 teaspoon ground allspice
3 tablespoons vegetable oil
2/3 cup dark molasses
1/4 cup honey
2 egg whites
2/3 cup plain, nonfat yogurt
1/2 cup golden raisins
Vegetable cooking spray
1 tablespoon powdered sugar (optional)

1. Stir all ingredients (except yogurt and raisins) together until just blended. Fold in yogurt and raisins.

2. Pour the batter into a 9-inch square nonstick baking pan coated with vegetable cooking spray.

3. Bake in a preheated 350°F oven for 25 to 30 minutes or until a wooden toothpick inserted in the center comes out clean.

4. Cool pan on a wire rack for 10 minutes; remove cake and transfer to serving plate.

5. Dust with powdered sugar (optional).

9 SERVINGS
230 CALORIES PER SERVING; 4.9 GRAMS OF FAT;
0.6 GRAM OF SATURATED FAT;
LESS THAN 1 MILLIGRAM OF CHOLESTEROL

Espresso Cake

1 cup cake flour
1 1/4 cup powdered sugar
12 large egg whites
4 tablespoons instant espresso granules
1 1/2 teaspoons cream of tartar
1/4 teaspoon salt
1 1/2 teaspoons vanilla extract
1 1/4 cups granulated sugar

Mocha Icing:
2 teaspoons instant espresso powder
3 teaspoons cocoa powder, divided
2 tablespoons hot water
1 1/2 cups powdered sugar

1. Sift cake flour and 1 1/4 cups of powdered sugar together in a small bowl. Set aside.

2. Place room temperature egg whites, espresso, cream of tartar, and salt in a large mixing bowl. Beat at high speed until soft peaks form.

3. Add vanilla and continue beating. Gradually incorporate granulated sugar, a few tablespoons at a time so that sugar can dissolve.

4. Keep beating at high speed until egg whites form stiff peaks; carefully fold in flour mixture.

5. Spoon batter into an ungreased 10-inch tube pan. Bake in a preheated 375°F oven for 35 to 40 minutes or until cake springs back when lightly touched. Invert pan and cool completely.

6. Loosen cake from sides of pan with a narrow metal spatula.

Espresso Cake, continued

Icing

1. Mix espresso powder and 1 teaspoon of cocoa powder into hot water until dissolved. Stir in 1 1/2 cups of powdered sugar.

2. Drizzle icing over cake; sprinkle with remaining cocoa powder.

....

12 SERVINGS
220 CALORIES PER SERVING; 0.1 GRAM OF FAT;
TRACE OF SATURATED FAT; 0 CHOLESTEROL

Papaya Sorbet

1 ripe papaya (1 1/4 pounds), diced
1/4 cup plain low-fat yogurt
1/2 cup light corn syrup
1 teaspoon fresh lime juice

....

1. Place papaya in a 9-inch square baking pan and freeze for about 1 hour

2. Place frozen papaya in food processor with yogurt, corn syrup, and lime juice. Process until smooth. Freeze for at least 1 hour. Makes 2 cups.

....

4 SERVINGS, 1/2 CUP EACH
160 CALORIES; 0 FAT; 1 MILLIGRAM OF CHOLESTEROL

Traditional Tapioca

2 tablespoons quick-cooking tapioca
3 tablespoons sugar
1/8 teaspoon salt
1 egg, beaten
2 cups skim milk
1/2 teaspoon vanilla

1. Mix all ingredients (except vanilla) in a saucepan. Let stand 5 minutes.

2. Bring to a full boil, stirring constantly. Remove from heat. Stir in vanilla.

3. Stir again after 20 minutes. Chill.

4 SERVINGS, ABOUT 1/2 CUP EACH
115 CALORIES PER SERVING; 1.5 GRAMS OF FAT;
0.5 GRAM OF SATURATED FAT; 55 MILLIGRAMS OF CHOLESTEROL

Harvest Apple Cake

4 cups (1 1/4 pounds) unpeeled, chopped
Golden Delicious apples, divided
1 cup firmly packed brown sugar
3/4 cup each all-purpose and whole wheat flour
1 teaspoon baking soda
1 teaspoon cinnamon
1/2 teaspoon salt
1/4 teaspoon each ginger and cloves
1/4 cup vegetable oil
2 large eggs, lightly beaten
1 teaspoon vanilla extract
1 tablespoon confectioners' sugar

1. Combine 3 cups of the apples and the sugar in a bowl; let stand 45 minutes.
2. Heat oven to 350°F. Grease and flour a 6-cup fluted tube pan.
3. Combine dry ingredients in a medium bowl. Combine oil, eggs, and vanilla in a small bowl; stir into the apple-sugar mixture. Stir in dry ingredients and remaining apples until blended.
4. Pour into the prepared pan. Bake 40 to 45 minutes, until a toothpick inserted in the center of cake comes out clean. Cool in the pan on a wire rack 10 minutes; unmold cake and cool completely. Sprinkle with confectioners' sugar.

12 SERVINGS
213 CALORIES PER SERVING; 6 GRAMS OF FAT;
1 GRAM OF SATURATED FAT; 35 MILLIGRAMS OF CHOLESTEROL

Peach Yogurt Pudding and Pie Filling

16-ounce can sliced peaches in light syrup
1 envelope unflavored gelatin
2 tablespoons sugar
1/3 cup frozen orange juice concentrate
1/16 teaspoon almond extract
1/4 teaspoon vanilla extract
8-ounce carton plain, low-fat yogurt

1. Drain and coarsely chop peaches; save 2/3 cup of the liquid.

2. Mix gelatin and sugar. Add peach liquid; heat, stirring constantly, until gelatin is dissolved.

3. Stir in orange juice concentrate and extracts. Chill until mixture has the consistency of egg white.

4. Whip until fluffy. Fold in yogurt and add peaches.

5. Pour into a pie shell. Chill until set.

8 SERVINGS, 1/8 OF 9-INCH PIE (FILLING ONLY)
OR 1/3 CUP SERVING OF PUDDING EACH
80 CALORIES PER SERVING; 0.5 GRAM OF FAT;
0.3 GRAM OF SATURATED FAT;
LESS THAN 5 MILLIGRAMS OF CHOLESTEROL

Extras

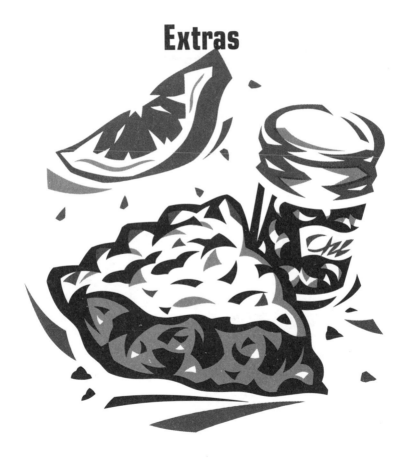

Skim the Fat

Pie Crust With Oil

1 cup whole wheat flour
1/2 teaspoon salt
2 tablespoons water
1/4 cup oil

1. Mix flour and salt thoroughly. Mix 3 tablespoons of the flour mixture with the water to make a paste.

2. Using a fork, lightly mix oil with remaining flour mixture until mixture is crumbly. Stir flour paste into flour-oil mixture to form a ball.

3. Roll dough between 2 sheets of wax paper until the dough is at least 1 inch wider all around than the pie pan. Remove top paper.

4. Invert pastry, paper side up, over pie pan. Peel off remaining paper. Fit carefully into pie pan, lifting edging as necessary to eliminate air bubbles. Trim off irregular edges of dough, leaving about 1/2 inch beyond rim of pan. Fold dough under to edge of pan.

5. Flute edge of dough with fingers or press lightly to pan using tines of fork. Prick bottom and side well with fork.

6. Bake at 450°F until lightly browned (about 11 minutes). Cool and fill as desired.

8 SERVINGS, 1/8 OF 9-INCH PIE CRUST
110 CALORIES PER SERVING; 7.1 GRAMS OF FAT;
0.9 GRAM OF SATURATED FAT; 0 CHOLESTEROL

Middle Eastern Bean Spread (Hummus)

16-ounce can garbanzo beans
3 cloves garlic, crushed
3 tablespoons lemon juice
2 teaspoons olive oil
1/2 teaspoon cumin
1 tablespoon chopped parsley
1 pound assorted raw vegetables, such as broccoli florets,
carrot and celery sticks, green pepper slices

1. Drain garbanzo beans, reserving 1/4 cup of the liquid.

2. Place beans, reserved liquid, and remaining ingredients (except parsley and raw vegetables) into a blender or food processor.

3. Blend until smooth. Place in a serving dish and garnish with parsley; chill.

4. Arrange raw vegetables on a platter; offer hummus as a dip. Spread hummus on bagels, pita bread, or sandwiches if desired.

12 SERVINGS, 2 TABLESPOONS EACH
55 CALORIES PER SERVING; 1.5 GRAMS OF FAT;
0.2 GRAM OF SATURATED FAT; 0 CHOLESTEROL

Peach Chutney

3 large peaches, peeled and diced
1/4 cup yellow pepper, diced
1/4 cup red onion, finely chopped
1/4 cup dates, chopped
3/4 cup frozen apple juice concentrate
2 tablespoons white vinegar
1 tablespoon fresh ginger, grated
1/2 teaspoon nutmeg
1/8 teaspoon crushed red pepper flakes

1. Place all ingredients in a deep 1 1/2-quart microwave container; mix gently.
2. Cook uncovered at full power for 7 minutes.
3. Refrigerate tightly covered until well chilled; keep for up to 1 week. Serve with grilled fish or meat, or spread onto sandwiches.

5 SERVINGS, ABOUT 1/2 CUP EACH
125 CALORIES PER SERVING; 0.4 GRAM OF FAT;
0.1 GRAM OF SATURATED FAT; 0 CHOLESTEROL

Mushroom Sauce

1 tablespoon margarine
1 1/2 tablespoons flour
1/4 teaspoon salt
3/4 cup skim milk
2-ounce can mushrooms, sliced and drained

1. Heat margarine; stir in flour and salt. Add milk slowly, stirring constantly; cook until thickened.
2. Add mushrooms and heat to serving temperature.

4 SERVINGS, ABOUT 1/4 CUP EACH
55 CALORIES PER SERVING; 3 GRAMS OF FAT;
0.6 GRAM OF SATURATED FAT; TRACE OF CHOLESTEROL

Mock Sour Cream

1/2 cup cottage cheese, uncreamed (dry)
1/4 cup buttermilk
1 tablespoon oil
1 teaspoon lemon juice
1/8 teaspoon salt

1. Put all ingredients into blender container; cover and blend until smooth.
2. Serve over baked potatoes or other vegetables.

ABOUT 2/3 CUP
20 CALORIES PER TABLESPOON; 1.4 GRAMS OF FAT;
0.2 GRAM OF SATURATED FAT; TRACE OF CHOLESTEROL

Lighter Condiments

Consider adding chutneys and sauces made with little or no fat to the kitchen cupboard. Most of these colorful but lean ingredients spice up the looks and flavor of light menus. The following all have less than 1 gram of fat per tablespoon.

barbecue sauce

chili sauce

cranberry-orange chutney

horseradish

catsup

Dijon mustard

pickle relish

seafood cocktail sauce

soy sauce

teriyaki sauce

Worcestershire sauce

Skim the Fat

Index

Index

Index